100 Questions & Answers About Anxiety

Khleber Chapman Attwell, MD, MPH
Assistant Clinical Professor of Psychiatry
NYU School of Medicine

JONES AND BARTLETT PUBLISHERS
Sudbury, Massachusetts
BOSTON   TORONTO   LONDON   SINGAPORE

World Headquarters
Jones and Bartlett
Publishers
40 Tall Pine Drive
Sudbury, MA 01776
info@jbpub.com
www.jbpub.com

Jones and Bartlett
Publishers Canada
6339 Ormindale Way
Mississauga, Ontario L5V 1J2
CANADA

Jones and Bartlett
Publishers International
Barb House, Barb Mews
London W6 7PA
UK

Jones and Bartlett's books and products are available through most bookstores and online booksellers. To contact Jones and Bartlett Publishers directly, call 800-832-0034, fax 978-443-8000, or visit our website www.jbpub.com.

Substantial discounts on bulk quantities of Jones and Bartlett's publications are available to corporations, professional associations, and other qualified organizations. For details and specific discount information, contact the special sales department at Jones and Bartlett via the above contact information or send an email to specialsales@jbpub.com.

Library of Congress Cataloging-in-Publication Data
Attwell, Khleber Chapman.
  100 questions & answers about anxiety / Khleber Chapman Attwell.— 1st ed.
    p. cm.
  ISBN 0-7637-2717-2 (pbk.)
  1. Anxiety—Miscellanea. 2. Anxiety—Treatment. I. Title: One hundred questions and answers about anxiety. II. Title.
  RC531.A88 2006
  616.85'22—dc22

                                                                          2005012151

The authors, editor, and publisher have made every effort to provide accurate information. However, they are not responsible for errors, omissions, or for any outcomes related to the use of the contents of this book and take no responsibility for the use of the products described. Treatments and side effects described in this book may not be applicable to all patients; likewise, some patients may require a dose or experience a side effect that is not described herein. The reader should confer with his or her own physician regarding specific treatments and side effects. Drugs and medical devices are discussed that may have limited availability controlled by the Food and Drug Administration (FDA) for use only in a research study or clinical trial. The drug information presented has been derived from reference sources, recently published data, and pharmaceutical research data. Research, clinical practice, and government regulations often change the accepted standard in this field. When consideration is being given to use of any drug in the clinical setting, the health care provider or reader is responsible for determining FDA status of the drug, reading the package insert, reviewing prescribing information for the most up-to-date recommendations on dose, precautions, and contraindications, and determining the appropriate usage for the product. This is especially important in the case of drugs that are new or seldom used.

Production Credits

Executive Publisher: Christopher Davis
Production Director: Amy Rose
Editorial Assistant: Kathy Richardson
Production Assistant: Alison Meier
Associate Marketing Manager: Laura Kavigian
Manufacturing Buyer: Therese Connell
Composition: Northeast Compositors
Cover Design: Kate Ternullo
Cover Images: © Tad Denson/Shutterstock, Inc., Ablestock, and Photodisc
Printing and Binding: Malloy, Inc
Cover Printing: Malloy, Inc

Printed in the United States of America
09 08 07 06 05   10 9 8 7 6 5 4 3 2 1

Dedication

To all who have known the haunting of terror,
or the heartbreak of loss.

For all who seek the refreshment of safety.

Contents

Preface

Many thoughts come to mind, thinking of the preface. I want you to know what a pleasure it has been to prepare this book for Jones and Bartlett as a publisher and for you as a reader. I cannot think of a better topic than anxiety, as we all have anxiety all the time as a function of our evolutionary hard wiring and as a mental phenomenon that we experience as emotion. The question is how much is normal? This book is about teasing those differences apart and about getting the right kind of help when the anxiety becomes too much.

More than anything, this book aims to make anxiety less shameful. So many of us are so anxious talking about anxiety! We often feel that in sharing some of our deeper thoughts or feelings, we might risk losing the love, affection, or esteem of those we depend on. Or we fear that we might feel a depth of discomfort that we might not otherwise have the tools to handle. Thus, like so many friends, family, colleagues, and fellow citizens, we tell ourselves to shut up and repackage those disturbing, seemingly forbidden thoughts and feelings back into some corner recess of our minds—hopefully forever. All too soon, these threatening thoughts and feelings return to the surface, and that uncomfortable anxiety rears its unwanted head again. This book deals with getting into those fears with the aim of managing and understanding them better, a process that shame and fear of stigma only impede. If you can talk about your anxiety, you can feel better. I hope this book helps many of you to take that leap of faith across the canyons of mistrust, isolation, and fear that have been put in place over the years.

I know this story backward and forward, not only from my own life experiences and life-changing reaction to good treatment, I know it because my patients tell me this story almost every day. I know how much better we feel when we are able to share our seemingly shameful reactions and experiences with a gifted clinician; I also know how much relief people get from the symptoms with which they present, the ultimate takehome of good treatment. I wish to thank every patient, friend, or family member who has ever felt safe enough to speak with me candidly about their experiences with anxiety. Without your trust, I would never have learned all that I have about the nature of anxiety and its inseparability from our lives and mental worlds.

Jones and Bartlett had the confidence to allow me to write this book as it came to my mind. I walked home from the office most evenings after signing the book contract thinking about whatever anxious phenomenon's residue was most in my mind after that day's work. I kept a log of questions that arose, and then when I had a chance, I dictated my answers while imagining at the same time that I was answering the question for a patient in the office. I have tried as much as possible to keep the answers simple, understandable, and in a brass-tacks tone.

The greatest strength of the book comes from the patients' commentary. I cannot thank enough Rick Sostchen and Selma Duckler, the two individuals who, through their sharing of their experiences of anxiety and its treatment, have modeled the very spirit of making deeper anxious life experiences more approachable. I asked each of them to respond with what first came to his or her mind that seemed useful to the potential reader. Their comments resulted, and I could not have found two more wonderful people with whom to collaborate. Their stories speak for themselves. The National Alliance for the Mentally Ill and the American Psychoanalytic Association were invaluable in helping me to locate two individuals who were willing to go on the record writing about their anxiety. Enjoy!

The New Yorker cartoons are designed to make the material easier to relate to. In no way are they intended to be insensitive to the horror of profound anxiety. Conversely, I have often found that some of the worst experiences can eventually be lightened or sweetened in some way through the use of humor. It is with a desire to use any tool that might help someone to deal with his or her anxiety that humor appears in this book in the context that it does. Thanks to Meredith Miller from the *New Yorker* for arranging permission.

Similarly, Marc Ramsey from Anxiety Disorders Association of America granted permission for the publication of the rating scales that you will find in the back part of the book. These rating scales can allow you to measure the degree of anxiety in your life and serve as an easy way to start a conversation with your health-care professional.

I especially want to thank the entire staff at Jones and Bartlett. Chris Davis took the bet on me as an author and shepherded me through the publication process. Kathy Richardson and Alison Meier made the editing and production possible! Thank you all for your patience.

It will not be lost on you from reading this book that I am a big believer in talking as a way to get help. Medications save lives routinely, and I am not the first psychiatrist to believe wholeheartedly in medication as a lifesaving and therapeutic tool in symptom reduction. I prescribe medication when it will provide genuine relief, and I am deeply indebted to the pharmaceutical industry for creating, researching, and producing many of the effective pharmacotherapies available today. All pharmacological interventions discussed in this book stem from my own experience working with patients, a decision made easier by my not receiving any financial contributions from any pharmaceutical company nor owning any stock in pharmaceutical companies.

At the same time, I have healthy respect for that which a pill will not cure. Here lies the strength and backbone of psychotherapy. I know that if a patient will ever be able to live without medication, then talking with a doctor, sometimes intensively and over many years, provides a major route to relief from anxiety. I believe, based on my experience working with patients in psychotherapy and psychoanalysis, that the talking cure is at the heart of deep respect for the individual experience. Tailoring a treatment to the exact nature of what may go along with an individual's symptoms involves a lot of talking, listening, and relating. My training as a psychoanalyst and my experiences as a patient in analysis for many years have allowed me to appreciate the depth of change that we can transform within ourselves when motivated to do so. For this wisdom, and for the doctors, teachers, and supervisors who have taught me, I am eternally grateful.

Finally, I wish to thank all of the colleagues, friends, and family who have supported me during this enterprise. You know who you are and how much your love means to me. Sharing this experience as it happened in real time gave me a wonderful supply of confidence to take the next steps. I wish especially to thank my wife, Elizabeth, for her unflagging respect for what matters most to me. In addition to all of her practical help and accommodation of schedule, her love has buoyed my life through the writing process. For that love, and for the quiet devotion of our black Lab, Sasha, who sat by my side, I am always mindful and deeply appreciative.

Chap Attwell, MD, MPH
New York City

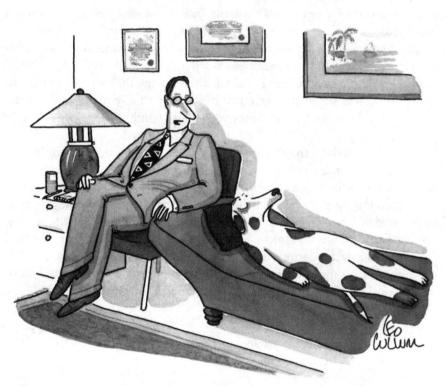

"You only <u>think</u> you're barking at nothing. We're <u>all</u> barking at <u>something</u>."

Reprinted with permission from The Cartoon Bank, a division of *The New Yorker* magazine.

Introduction

Welcome to *100 Questions & Answers About Anxiety*. This book, divided into three parts, answers the common questions about anxiety. Part I explores the nature of anxiety. Part II identifies the many faces of anxiety—from its normal, adaptive role to its ability to shape our personalities to its full-blown, recognizable disorders. In this second part, you read about the major ways in which anxiety might show up in a person's life, as well as some common manifestations of anxiety that you might recognize in yourself or in those close to you. In Part III, itself divided into three subsections, I explore treatment options: psychotherapy, pharmacotherapy, and other/alternative treatments for anxiety.

Finally, the book includes a glossary of basic terms important to an understanding of anxiety states; basic screening scales for anxiety disorders; and an appendix with references/resources useful in obtaining the appropriate health care you may need. You will be able to educate yourself further about anxiety and its nature and about the potential effect of this condition on you or your family.

Through its simulation of an educational consultation in the office of a working psychiatrist, the book intends to serve as a road map for understanding the shape of basic anxiety disorders and/or manifestations of clinical anxiety. It will help you distinguish normal, reactive anxiety from that which might overburden you and which may respond to treatment. You will get to know some of the anxiety syndromes by reading dozens of clinical vignettes—condensed and disguised—from numerous patients' lives. These stories, by design, capture the flavor of a symptom that you might experience. The book in no way serves as a replacement for seeking appropriate professional help. While certain references may be made to findings from neuroscience (brain chemistry and function), this text, in its heart, intends to focus on common clinical pictures seen on a daily basis in the office. The inclusion of personal reflection and commentary by Mr. Rick Sostchen and Ms. Selma Duckler distinguishes this book from other works on anxiety. Paying close attention to these patients' comments (responses to the text) will help you to gain a sense of what can happen in the understanding and treatment of anxiety and to overcome any fear you may have about seeking the appropriate kind of referral for yourself.

I am a clinician—a board-certified psychiatrist working mainly in private practice in New York City. I am also a psychoanalyst, recently having completed six years of adult psychoanalytic training and beginning several more ahead of child and adolescent psychoanalytic training. I have found the utility of this discipline and training indispensable. As much as I enjoy reading and learning about neuroscience, I am neither a basic scientist nor a clinical researcher. Any included references to neuroscience are intended only to deepen an understanding of any given person's symptoms.

In Part II, you will read about some of the infinite ways in which anxiety can affect a life. I have reviewed the kinds of anxiety I see most frequently in my practice or saw most regularly when I worked at Bellevue Hospital, in one of the busiest psychiatric emergency rooms in the country. The first part of this section addresses common questions, while the later part details some of the particular anxiety syndromes recognized by the *Diagnostic and Statistical Manual of Mental Disorders*.[1] Due to the staggering diversity of presentations of the same "anxiety disorder," I have included only examples that occur commonly. Please refer to the Rating Scales section in the back of the book if you believe you have one of the particular disorders. You can fill out the form and take it to your physician, who can make an appropriate psychiatric referral. It is essential that you not attempt to diagnose yourself or treat yourself without the help of a skilled professional, for reasons that will become clear.

Good treatment and choosing the right treatment for your personality style and your condition serve as the cornerstones of successful recovery. The adage "diagnosis before treatment" from the practice of medicine guides this choice. Obtaining a correct diagnosis can cost both time and money, but it is worth every minute and dollar, as the decisions made at this juncture can shape the course of the rest of your life. When you think about the money and time you spend looking into the feasibility and safety of buying your new home, it makes you realize that considering the repair of your internal home merits at least the same attention to detail. Many patients have reported that in the long run, the cost of their treatment was the best financial investment of their lives, as good treatment allowed them to advance professionally. Hence, minute for minute and dollar for dollar, they became more efficient and calmer within their own skin, making actual cost of treatment less of a cost than an investment in good troubleshooting. When people feel better, they make better decisions, have fewer health problems, better tolerate the health problems they already have, get along better with their families, fight less with their spouses or partners, abuse drugs less, and earn more money. One good decision can lead to many future good ones, and finding a reliable mental health professional—like finding the right cardiovascular surgeon—is serious business. The difference can literally be lifesaving.

Note

1. American Psychiatric Association. (2000). *Diagnostic and statistical manual of mental disorders* (4th ed., text revision). Washington, DC: American Psychiatric Association.

PART ONE

The Basics

What is anxiety?

What is the general philosophy of this book?

What is the difference between anxiety and fear?

More ...

1. What is anxiety?

We all have to make sense of what any given anxious moment may or may not mean. I go about this process in my office by taking the "anxiety temperature," as if on a thermometer (see Table 1). I visualize this instrument as being a basic warning scale that human beings use as part of our "fight-or-flight" survival response to

Table 1. Thermometer of anxiety.

Cooler	Warm	Hot
Most consciously in control; most repression of unconscious	*Still consciously in control, but with greater unconscious contribution*	*Less consciously in control; more unconscious contribution*
Mind	Mind	Mind
calm	keyed up	terrorized
carefree	worried	dread
integrated	stressed	overwhelmed
safe	tense	flooded
	sad	near death
	angry	racing thoughts
	lonely	
	empty	
	hurting	
	needy	
Body	Body	Body
normal heart rate	jittery	heart palpitations
breathing calmly	increased heart rate	sweating
able to concentrate	breathing faster	nausea/vomiting
not sweating	thinking faster, harder to concentrate	chest pain
	or	back pain
	back pain	dizziness
	abdominal pain	fainting
	headache/migraine	voice changes
	mild dizziness	shortness of breath
	diarrhea	
	constipation	

any potentially life-threatening situation. For example, if someone has a very high anxiety temperature, he perceives himself to be in real danger regardless of the actual circumstances. He might have some classic physiologic and/or psychological symptoms, which can feel above and beyond one's **conscious** control. He might experience characteristic chest pain, nausea, sweating, dizziness, and palpitations of the heart consistent with a **panic attack** at this high temperature. He also might have the psychological symptoms of intense worry, or of a sense of doom—that he could die or that some disaster will soon happen. This **fear** could become an obsessive worry about the magnitude of any given action in that moment. These types of symptoms would be diagnosable, in a formal kind of way, in the ***Diagnostic and Statistical Manual of Mental Disorders (DSM)***,[1] a descriptive field guide to the most commonly recognized psychiatric syndromes encountered today.

When our own or the patient's temperature is medium-high, we meet the types of daily, potentially less symptomatic, more potentially adaptive roles of anxiety. These states might belong more to a person's character, or to the way he or she has evolved over time. If our friends and family would characterize us as chronically anxious, we are likely in this range. Loneliness, dependency, anger, sadness, fear, or just needing to be in control of a situation might be related to anxiety. These feeling states may, in turn, be intimately connected to a behavior designed to respond to the given anxiety, which then defines itself, over time, as a character trait. Loneliness might lead to substance abuse; anger might lead to **aggression**; or dependency might lead to clinging. These less acute states may still

Conscious
thinking that is in one's awareness.

Panic attack
a severe anxiety attack that involves multiple symptoms, including extreme fear, trouble breathing, increased heart rate, sweating, and shakes.

Fear
an uncomfortable state of feeling, associated with anxiety, that something bad will or might happen.

DSM
the *Diagnostic and Statistical Manual*. This book contains a listing of all of the identified psychiatric diagnoses and their symptoms.

Aggression
a natural human emotion that involves angry, sometimes violent, ideas or behaviors.

3

impact a life substantially, however. Later, I will explain the potential benefits of treatment for this kind of seemingly less overt anxiety.

Finally, at the lower, cooler temperature ranges, one might be described as or simply feel free, carefree, euphoric, joyous, happy, relaxed, at peace, or calm—the feeling that life is safe and potentially going well at that moment, and that no immediate danger is at hand.

2. What is the general philosophy of this book?

Over the centuries much has been written on anxiety from many wide-ranging disciplines, including, but not limited to history, literature, biology, sociology, philosophy, and religion. All perspectives have attempted to wrestle with the question of anxiety, a basic question of existence. This book provides one person's cumulative experience treating and attempting to understand anxiety. In addition, this text aims to help you understand more about anxiety by sharing what I have found to be both common and helpful working with and puzzling over anxiety. I cannot claim more of the truth than any other discipline, but I do hope to provide a sense of what goes through my mind in my office when I attempt to help a patient with anxiety.

Any patient material that I might use in the book is entirely composite; it in no way portrays one particular patient. All of the syndromes and examples used illustrate general principles that occur time and time again in the office, just as an internist deals repeatedly with chest pain and shortness of breath. If there is any particular point in the material where a footnote or reference might be useful, I will mention the author and the name of the book and/or article. However, most of the information in the book is widely available both in common textbooks on anxiety or on the World Wide Web. Any particular information quoted is part of the public domain unless otherwise noted; all other individual perspectives are mine, stemming from the aggregate years of discussion and thinking with colleagues and patients about these matters.

3. What is the difference between anxiety and fear?

The difference between anxiety and fear is an important distinction. Anxiety serves as the body's warning system—the brain's way of telling the body that something bad *could* happen. This response relates to but is distinct from fear, which alarms us when something actually dangerous is happening or is just about to happen. For example, if you become scared that you will lose your spouse from medical illness in anticipation of his routine medical checkup, in the absence of any known medical condition, this reaction would be considered anxiety about losing your spouse. The reasons for this anxiety are very important; you may well have suffered from some prior significant loss and/or trauma. In turn, the fear that this trauma could recur ("once bitten, twice shy") might cause your anxiety that something bad might or will happen again. This situation—anxiety—would differ from someone who lives with a spouse with metastatic cancer. In this situation,

The Basics

5

the patient's spouse will die, even if the right treatment is provided; it is simply a matter of when the emotional pain and loss will occur. In this situation, fear of the spouse's dying—with its host of mental and physical reactions—would be entirely appropriate and in keeping with reality.

This example highlights the essential interface between anxiety and fear and underscores the historical origins of any particular individual's anxiety. Most of the time, people seem to become anxious about events in the present based, in part, upon genuinely fearful situations from their past. The fear of today can lead to the anxiety of tomorrow. This phenomenon allows us to think about anxiety as a form of remembering prior traumas, losses, or significant life events (see question 15).

Rick's comments:

I remember reading a quote from Mark Twain, I believe it was, who wrote that the worst things in his life never happened. Anxiety sufferers such as me know what Mr. Twain means. The time and attention I give to possible negative outcomes and events—to things that have little likelihood of happening—is all out of proportion to the time and attention they deserve. The waste of energy is enormous! Plus, it means I'm spending less time either doing things that could actually be productive or taking an action that could help me avoid some real, not phantom, difficulties.

4. What is the difference between normal and pathologic anxiety?

Pathologic
this refers to any medical condition that is considered abnormal.

Using the thermometer in Table 1 as a metaphor for understanding normal versus **pathologic** anxiety, one might consider normal anxiety as that which keys the body and prompts us to action in a way that helps us function better in life. Pathologic anxiety would prevent someone from doing what she wishes to do or from feeling how she would like to feel. For example, an upcoming test or performance can motivate us to study or prepare for the challenge at hand. However, when pathological, this anxiety might drift into obsessing on all of the details necessary to prepare for the test but never actually preparing. Writers, musicians, or students display this anxiety via procrastination, postponing aspects of their preparation out of a sense of fear. This stalling can subsequently mushroom in time to a mental and physical paralysis, thus leaving them unable to perform in the originally desired fashion. All anxiety, pathologic or normal, serves as an important communication of a feeling which can be used to help us perceive more precisely what stimulus in our environments might trigger our fear. Paying close attention can help us better distinguish the nature of the fear, and thereby respond more appropriately (less pathologically).

5. What is the difference between conscious and unconscious anxiety?

Conscious anxiety is that which we know we fear. Snakes, heights, germs, a first date, a big presentation, taking a test, or going to the doctor are all common conscious fears. **Unconscious** anxiety is that which is beyond our conscious awareness. This anxiety most often declares itself when someone has a panic attack seemingly out of the blue. The person might say that he is "freaking out" but cannot say what the trigger was. Perhaps he was driving home for Christmas and harbored deep, unconscious resentment at his family's rejection of his partner but was not able to know consciously at that time that this distress was at the root of

Unconscious
the thought processes of which one is not aware.

7

the panic attack. The two—conscious and unconscious awareness—can also go together. A person can tell you he is afraid of blood but be less able to tell you that he hates blood because it reminds him of the death of his mother years ago when she went to the hospital bleeding. Or, a woman may fear blood because of her or her mother's not knowing how to handle her first period. Now he or she consciously fears losing his or her spouse from an accident but cannot tolerate that idea or feeling and so avoids these partially conscious fears and focuses consciously instead on hating avoiding blood.

Rick's comments:

My anxiety disorder is obsessive-compulsive disorder (OCD). I find that my anxiety is provoked by both fears I know I have and ones of which I'm not even aware. When I'm facing something that makes me nervous, like a doctor's visit or an unexpected bill, the symptoms of my OCD intensify. For example, I might say, either out loud or to myself, phrases or thoughts which I repeat endlessly. Or I might feel the need to touch something (the T.V. detective Monk, a fellow, if fictional, OCD sufferer does this, too). Or I might avoid certain words and numbers or combinations of numbers (such as but, 4, *or numbers totaling 18). Or I might replay in my mind an old argument I've had with someone. Sometimes these and other symptoms pop up even when I am not confronted with something that I know makes me anxious. Maybe when I have nothing to worry about, I find that relaxation something to worry about!*

Selma's comments:

When I started analysis, I believed in the unconscious when I read about it. I was reading Freud's Interpretation of Dreams, but I actually didn't believe it pertained to me. I believed in my ability to exercise willpower and the poem by William Henley that most spoke to me, Invictus, ended with, "I am the master of my fate; I am the captain of my soul." At that time, I believed conscious willpower was the only way to achieve mastery of my fate. Of course, I always failed. But I always started again, with what I thought each time to be more willpower. Freud's delightful idea of the unconscious, so attractive on the printed page, I didn't hold to have much to do with me.

In all the years of my treatment, evidence of unconscious activity, both desirable and very much undesirable, consistently appeared, no matter what I called it (and I never—ever—called it unconscious drive). I had all kinds of names for it however, and frequently in the beginning years, I decided I did these undesirable things because of my analysts. I thought that through his suggestion he made me do them! It took a long time for me to really understand that what I did came out of my head and from my needs and feelings. It took even longer (in years, not months) to have respect for that process and to not invest so much in my willpower that, for sure, put all the things I didn't want to do into great activity. Eventually I learned that I put in place my excessive attempts at willpower because of my very strong feelings that exactly the opposite should happen.

For example, I always dieted. I considered myself very fat, and if I were up a pound, I would frequently not continue on with my social plans, being so ashamed of my ballooned look. In actuality, I weighed 112 pounds at 5 feet, 4 inches. I had great willpower (which also broke) and had so many restrictions that I felt were life-giving. Breaking one food restriction meant falling into chaos. It took me a long time to know (not know in my head, but in my gut) that I needed all these intense restrictions because of a tremendous

The Basics

9

desire to eat. I was never actually hungry, so this realization was very hard for me to figure out. More than that, I negated at every possibility what this desire to eat meant to me until there was no turning away. I had to accept my persistent desire to return to an infantile state. Psychologically for me, all else represented a separation from this feeling of being taken care of that I could experience only as death. I could not turn away from this knowledge because its evidence was so present in my life, and not always consciously. I saw supremely strong signs of active, demanding, powerful, heretofore unconscious activity that in this example shaped my eating anxieties and all of the energy I spent in their management.

As my treatment deepened, I was more able to use my beloved willpower as a conscious application to my unconscious drives, which I then accepted as a real part of me. For example, I used the public library extensively, as I loved to read. It was available and accessible, and my books were always overdue. I had library fines of $30 and upwards. One day, I griped about them in a session, and then quickly went on to more seemingly pressing, important problems. My analyst wanted to go back to the library fines—why were they so high? I retorted that with all of my problems, library fines were no significant place to work. I went back to the serious, upsetting problems. And back he returned to the library fines. This back and forth repeated, and I became very angry. Finally I jumped up from the couch and said that if he was concerned about my library fines when I had real problems, then he was crazy and certainly couldn't help me. I did not know what I was doing there and stormed out. I intended to end the analysis.

I came back the next day, not apologetic, and not subdued. But at least I was willing to see this thing through. In time (and I don't mean by that afternoon), I could see that returning the books on time contained for me a deep sense of separation that I couldn't tolerate. These books gave me such joy and told me in every way stories of life and how to live life; they provided a great loving, substitute mother. Was I going to return the books and give that up? Never.

When these notions took root in my head, the overdue books trick never worked for me again. It was over. In the end, the gift to me wasn't that I no longer had library fines, but rather that I understood a little bit more about what I was doing with my life. One little piece of deep knowledge all of a sudden opened other doors, and I could see similar behavior in so many other areas of my life. I didn't even have to think about it or make an effort. The patterns that no longer worked for me disappeared. I wasn't playing those games anymore. I began to use my energies in much more creative ways.

6. What are life's normal, expected phases of anxiety?

Normal, adaptive anxiety is a feature inherent to human development. As we progress from one stage to the next, we have to experience anxiety to get from point A to point B. Austrian neurologist Sigmund Freud used the birth of the infant as a model for explaining what might happen in understanding anxiety. He saw us—like the baby leaving the womb—as leaving one comfortable place to enter a new place, though less comfortable initially despite its also affording greater freedom. With each developmental phase, new anxieties appear; we have to prepare for the next step towards autonomy. Children learn to walk and to separate from their parents. In American culture, we often leave home to go to school or to college. Or, as we become sexually active, choose a long-term mate, entertain the complexities of parenthood, navigate the vicissitudes of normal aging, or cope with medical illness or death, we relive the built-in human experience of anxiety about what might happen in the next phase. Moving to the next phase provides the desired liberation from the constraints of the prior phase or a feared loss of those freedoms in the case of end-of-life stages.

These anxious phases are all within the normal range. In any given life, one phase's progress may resonate with a particular person's experience from a prior phase. For example, a child who suffers from early parental divorce or parental loss from illness may have a harder time leaving home and being independent due to painful memories or fears. A child might feel responsible for the caretaking of the remaining parent or feel that her leaving home might kill that parent, whom she also loves and needs. These fears could resonate with actual feelings stirred in association to the divorce, when people who are significant to the child's world did leave and did cause pain.

Rick's comments:

Freud's definitely onto something—I was doing just fine in the womb. Since then, things have gotten shakier. I'm aware that I have avoided potentially enjoyable, worthwhile, and important activities because of anxiety—either because of fear of failure or just plain fear. This is where anxiety has not served a useful function. Instead of helping me to avoid danger, it whispers that life is dangerous so avoid, avoid, avoid . . . On the more positive side, when I don't let anxiety and OCD prevent me from doing something new and exciting, I have a real feeling of accomplishment.

7. *What questions can I ask myself about my anxiety to understand it better?*

a. Is this symptom new in onset or more longstanding (i.e., what is my history with this particular symptom?)

b. Is this symptom present more in my mind (e.g., worry) or in my body (e.g., nausea)?

c. How high is the temperature on the anxiety thermometer?

d. When I have had these symptoms before, what has helped me?

e. What kind of treatment does my doctor think would help me the most (short-term versus long-term, dynamic versus behavioral, medication versus not, **psychiatrist** versus **psychologist** or social worker, symptom focus versus personality focus)?

f. How much does substance abuse complicate my condition and/or improvement?

g. What makes my symptoms get better or worse during this episode?

h. Who else in my family has any symptom like this and what has helped them get better, or what has made them worse?

i. What does this particular symptom mean to me?

j. How much of my anxiety comes from feeling alone or unable to cope by myself, and how much of it comes from feeling that what I feel will be unacceptable to others (i.e., they would leave me if they knew what I was really feeling)?

The Basics

**Psychiatry/
psychiatrist**

the study, diagnosis, treatment, and prevention of mental illness and behavioral disorders. Psychiatrists are medical doctors (MDs) who study and practice psychiatry.

**Psychology/
psychologist**

the study of behavior and the processes underlying behavior. Psychologists are those who specialize in the study of psychology and have acquired their PhDs.

8. How common are anxiety disorders?

The statistics of anxiety disorder cases are difficult to determine with precision, and different sources cite different percentages (see David H. Barlow's book[2] for detailed discussion). However, in multiple transcultural, international studies, it appears that at any given point in time anywhere from 2 to 17% of the population may have one or more diagnosable anxiety disorders, including generalized anxiety disorder, posttraumatic stress disorder, obsessive-compulsive disorder, panic disorder, **agoraphobia**, simple phobia, or social phobia. Over a lifetime, that can translate into a 10 to 25% prevalence of diagnosable anxiety disorders before adding to that list those suffering from substance abuse disorders, apparent medical problems largely attributable to anxiety, or chronic anxiety that has become a core feature of a personality. As we examine the many faces of anxiety in general and focus on some of these syndromes in particular, I will highlight wherever possible the most recent estimates of the prevalence of any given syndrome in the U.S. population. For example, Table 2 references estimated prevalence of anxiety disorders in the United States.

Agoraphobia

a fear of open spaces or places from which escape might be difficult or help unavailable.

9. Why is anxiety so confusing to make sense of?

An understanding of anxiety often eludes us because it is so multifaceted, and you will discover how complex many of these faces can be in the next section. This process can be so confusing precisely because it is so normal to maintain a certain degree of anxiety, just as we all need a certain blood pressure in order to maintain consciousness. Like blood pressure, anxiety is nec-

Table 2   Estimated Prevalence of Anxiety Disorders in the United States

Anxiety Disorder	Estimated Prevalence Rates*	Question Number in this book
Generalized Anxiety Disorder	2–8%	60
Panic Disorder	1–4%	65
Social Phobia	2–15%	63
Specific Phobia	10%	64
Obsessive-Compulsive Disorder	2–3%	62
Post-Traumatic Stress Disorder	2–15%	66
Body Dysmorphic Disorder	1–2.2% (6–15% in dermatology and cosmetic surgery clinics)	55
Hypochondriasis	1.1–4.5%	61

*From Kaplan and Sadock's Comprehensive Textbook of Psychiatry

essary for our survival. Anxiety can also present as a subpiece of many different clinical pictures, thus making it a challenge to distinguish what is primarily anxiety and what is primarily another mental disorder with an anxious feature. For example, a provider never knows when initially treating someone dependent on alcohol how much internal anxiety serves as the primary driving force behind her alcoholism. **Depression**, manic depression, or a genetic predisposition to addiction and alcoholism can serve equally as motivations for drinking. In a classic example, a patient might present to the office complaining of overwhelming anxiety and panic attacks but also experience a psychotic break with reality consistent with a first onset of schizophrenia. Understandably, the feeling of losing your mind—knowing that your mind does not work as before—can produce anxiety that feels overwhelming. However,

Depression

a mood state in which one has numerous symptoms, including sleep and appetite disturbances, a decrease in energy level, concentration and interest, a feeling of sadness or isolation, and sometimes, thoughts of suicide.

The Basics

anxiety would not be the primary illness at hand, though it would be a critical component of the picture.

Rick's comments:

Because I am coping with depression as well as with OCD, I do find it difficult to figure out which causes which, if, in fact, one diagnosis has led to the other. Certainly, being depressed at times could have triggered my desire for greater control over my environment, which OCD provides at least the illusion of achieving. On the other hand, not being able to leave my bed without repeating a particular phrase first, or doing so with a series of words that cycle and recycle in my head from the moment I've woken up can be depressing. I'm trying to control things by doing something that makes me feel totally out of control! On the other hand . . . well, it's confusing. If I had to guess, I would say that the depression came first, however I wouldn't be surprised if I simultaneously also had OCD, too, without realizing it, or recognizing the symptoms at that time as being symptoms.

10. How can the human mind ward off anxiety?

One of the major contributions of the psychoanalytic school of thought from the last hundred years has been a detailed analysis of ways in which we deal with the discomfort of anxiety. Sometimes called **defense mechanisms**, these intrapsychic maneuvers serve to manage the tides of anxiety in our minds and bodies. In Freud's classic formulation, outlined in *Inhibitions, Symptoms, and Anxiety,*[3] he details the way in which the body reacted to a perceived danger as being signal anxiety. This reaction signaled the mind to engage in

Defense mechanism

a method of preventing harmful emotions from being felt.

16

defense against the obnoxious feeling by seeking a solution. Freud focused on repression (the unconscious **denial** of an uncomfortable stimulus), while his daughter, Anna, detailed many of the defense mechanisms in her classic work, *The Ego and the Mechanisms of Defense.*[4] She classified, for example, such mechanisms as isolation of feeling (distancing oneself from the painful feelings of a story), displacement (putting the blame onto something or someone outside of oneself, seen in kicking a dog or fearing a tunnel), or **somatization** (converting what would otherwise be overwhelming conscious feelings into bodily experiences). Today, often categorized on a spectrum from less to more mature in nature, the work of George Vaillant in *Adaptation to Life*[5] has helped us to understand that some defensive styles work much better than others in dealing with anxiety. More primitive styles include the use of projection and splitting (dividing the world into black and white, seeing someone or oneself as all good or all bad, or attributing one's own badness to those around him), while more successful styles involve the use of sublimation, altruism, or humor (using one's own history of trauma to better society or to make people laugh).

Vaillant's work suggests that in any given lifetime, a certain amount of calamity will invariably occur. Based on our own defensive styles, he suggests that it is not what happens to us in our lifetime that matters as much as how we choose to deal with it. He underscores one of the hallmarks of any good therapy for anxiety: helping the patient to see that making the lemon into lemonade or finding a way to see the glass as half full is a choice that remains in our control.

Denial
a particular defense mechanism that involves a refusal to believe that something is true.

Ego
one of three theoretical parts of the mind, first established by Sigmund Freud, that involves a person's ability to interact with reality, regulate mood, and participate in normal daily interactions.

Somatization
a process by which a person expresses emotional discomfort, most commonly anxiety, in the form of somatic, or bodily, symptoms.

The Basics

While anxiety may be inevitable and desirable for survival, using it to our advantage maximally will help us to function more highly.[5]

11. What is the neurobiology of anxiety?

The 20th century was a watershed in neurobiology; in particular, the years 1990 to 2000 were the "decade of the brain." To understand the neurobiology of anxiety comprehensively would require an intensive familiarity with **neurochemistry** and neuroanatomy. The reader might enjoy taking a look at Joseph LeDoux's *The Emotional Brain*, in which a wonderful illustration of the emotional circuitry of the brain becomes intimately connected to the way we perceive fear. LeDoux details the different inputs, conscious and unconscious, from an immediate sensory input (sight and smell) to higher thinking ("this is a stick, not a snake") and examines their creation, neuroanatomically, of our emotional and bodily flight-or-fight response.[6]

Several basic things show up time and again in today's research, all of which make our work very exciting and gratifying in 2005. We know certain areas of the brain axis are highly involved in the creation of anxiety. In particular, a region called the **amygdala** responds to potentially dangerous stimuli by chemically arousing the body to respond immediately. When danger is perceived to be close at hand, the amygdala's connections to the rest of the body bypass any areas of higher thought, which make our bodies respond in a fight-or-flight way. This circuitry (called the **limbic system**, as in liminal, or threshold between emotion and thought), in turn, makes the memory of the particular

Neurochemistry
the study of the mechanisms and chemical components of the nervous system, including brain structure and neurotransmitter function.

Amygdala
a part of the limbic system of the brain that is involved with learning, coordination of sensory input, and emotions.

Limbic system
the part of the brain that controls emotional responses and experiences.

trauma or perceived trauma indelible and codes the input of this memory on file for use in future dangerous situation assessments. We know that chronic **stress** is associated with an increase in **cortisol**, which can result in the creation of illness or have all kinds of deleterious long-term effects on the body, making the expense of long-term anxiety quite costly to the body (in extreme panic, cortisol can flood the body and create a shock similar to surgical shock, or sudden death).

Panic disorder and posttraumatic stress disorders are the best studied in the neurobiological realm; however, many exciting areas remain for future discovery with respect to **imaging** and understanding the roles of all of the different **neurotransmitters** which the brain uses in its regulation of anxiety. Major neurotransmitters that receive frequent mention include cortisol, epinephrine, **norepinephrine, γ-aminobutyric acid (GABA)**, and **serotonin**. It is just as important to remember that literally hundreds of unidentified neurotransmitters make up the complexity of our thinking and feelings, as well as their connections to the rest of the body. While we may know something about the actions of any given neurotransmitter, it is still too early to know how those interactions may cascade or interface downstream with the entire "soup" of our brain chemistry.

Rick's comments:

In the answer to Question 10, it is mentioned that one successful style of dealing with anxiety is humor. I've performed and written some comedy, so this seems to apply. I bring this up a question later because my first reaction to LeDoux's example of higher thinking ("this is a stick, not

The Basics

Stress

a general term to describe any event or situation that raises a person's anxiety.

Cortisol

a hormone secreted by the adrenal gland in response to stressful situations, including anxiety, fear, excitement and physical stress.

Imaging

the process of looking at parts of the human body that cannot be seen from the outside. Examples include x-rays, CAT scans and MRIs.

Neurotransmitter

a chemical messenger in the nervous system that carries a message from one neuron to the next. Examples include serotonin and norepinephrine.

Norepinephrine

a neurotransmitter (chemical) that helps regulate mood and other physical symptoms of anxiety.

19

GABA

Gamma-*aminobu-tyric acid*. A neurotransmitter in the central nervous system that is primarily involved in inhibiting impulses.

Serotonin

a neurotransmitter (chemical) in the central nervous system that is involved in many different activities, including motor function, mood regulation, and perception.

a snake") was: "wasn't that the mistake that Yul Brenner made in the movie The Ten Commandments?" When I am doing something that causes me anxiety (writing, for instance) I am more likely to think in humorous or offbeat ways. When, as a youngster, some friends and I walked on a frozen lake, which terrified me, I was actually coming up with one joke after another to hide my fear. (The next time you see someone standing on a frozen lake doing a comedy routine, it's probably me.) Now that's neurobiology!

12. What is the relationship between gender and anxiety?

Anxiety-related gender differences are complicated. In general, for reasons that seem entirely unknown to researchers at this time, women appear to be twice as likely as men either to inherit and/or experience an anxiety disorder, wherever they are in the world and regardless of treatment status. One obvious difference is biology: female versus male hormones. Does the presence of estrogen somehow sensitize women to a heightened sense of panic, perhaps useful in an evolutionary way to protect the nest? Cultural factors commonly appear as other sources of causation, looking at worldwide patterns in which it appears more socially acceptable for women and girls to experience fear as a symptom and to seek relief for it, while men and boys are more conditioned to avoid any display of this fear, or to counter it with reactive types of denial. Hence, men afraid of destruction may become hunters; men afraid to show pain may actively deny it when in the hospital. Finally, it seems more likely that men may experience just as much anxiety as women but choose to deal with it in what they perceive to be more socially acceptable ways, such as substance abuse or violence.

13. What is the relationship between temperament, genetics, and anxiety?

All of our symptoms occur within a human body. Inasmuch as the human body is genetic and comprised of **DNA** from each of our parents, there are dispositions towards the creation of anxiety that are inherited, just as with dispositions toward the creation of blood pressure or blood sugar in the clinical abnormalities of hypertension or diabetes.

I will not focus on the specifics of any genetic disorder involved in anxiety other than to say that population studies indicate that anxiety disorders tend to run in families and that researchers cannot find any single gene responsible for any given anxiety disorder. Anxiety appears to run along the more polygenic model, meaning that multiple **genes** and interactions between gene products create the states that go along with anxiety. This pattern makes the visible genetic picture (**phenotype**) of any given inherited gene structure (**genotype**) malleable, both to its environmental stimuli and its random interplay of inherited gene products.

Environmental interactions can shape any given clinical symptom, much as any organism in biology has its niche. For example, we know that identical twins (from one egg) separated at birth have a higher tendency to have anxiety disorders than fraternal twins (from two eggs) separated at birth. We know that children who have a shy **temperament** have a higher

The Basics

DNA
Deoxyribonucleic acid. The building block of all living creatures, it is a helical arrangement of proteins that carries one's genetic code.

Genes
packets of DNA, located on the chromosomes in each living cell of the human body, that carry all the information about how any given cell is supposed to function.

Phenotype
the physical representation of a particular genetic code (genotype).

Genotype
the particular set of genes that a person has for a particular trait or feature.

Temperament
the style of interaction and attachment with which a person is naturally born.

21

degree of anxiety disorders in life than children who have an outgoing disposition. However, we also know that a shy child who grows up in a more gregarious household learns that social interaction can be a safe medium of exchange. These findings suggest that the genetic template of any given person is malleable, based upon the environment in which a child grows up or in which an adult lives or receives treatment. Furthermore, we know that patients with anxiety disorders get better in **psychotherapy**, meaning that whatever given phenotype of illness they may walk in the door with, they are likely to leave with a different, less intense expression of anxiety. All of these data suggest that the clinical manifestation of anxiety is not unilaterally determined by any person's genetic structure.

Psychotherapy

a general term to describe many different types of psychological and psychiatric treatments that involve communication and talking between the patient and the therapist.

14. Can a medical illness or a drug reaction make me anxious?

It is important always to keep in mind that medical abnormalities can present as anxiety disorders. This principle proves critical to establishing the correct diagnosis. Much as a patient with physical symptoms may feel his problem is not psychiatric, so, too, can a patient with anxiety and worry not feel that her problems could be medical. The most classic example of this would be a woman who presents with new onset anxiety but has an overactive thyroid. It could also be a man who cannot explain his new onset panic attacks but neglects to mention his recent experimentation with cocaine. Another example would be a man who did not put together his heightened anxiety in crowds and while taking tests with his prior accident, when he went through the windshield of the car and sustained a concussion. A woman who cannot pinpoint the onset of her irritability to the starting of birth control pills or the onset of menopause is another example. This could also occur in the case of an elderly gentleman who becomes anxious about not being able to concentrate on his job but neglects to tell his doctor about his history of promiscuity and turns out to have untreated syphilis. Epilepsy, new-onset cancers, or HIV can have their first manifestations be psychiatric in nature.

Always keeping a watchful eye on what might be a psychiatric manifestation of a medical problem can prove invaluable in the long run and allow a therapist to direct the patient in the right direction. We cannot separate the brain and its health from the body and its conditions. Therefore, it does not surprise us that women who drink while they are pregnant predispose their infants to a wide range of developmental, learning, and/or psychiatric vulnerability. This principle also means that even if your mental health care provider is a physician, you would do well to check in with your primary care provider.

Rick's comments:

While I don't doubt that a medical illness can have a "psychiatric manifestation," I'm also aware that many of us who have a diagnosis of mental illness are wary and even angered when we feel that our physical symptoms are too easily discounted as being "all in our heads." The concern is that when a medical chart indicates that an individual has had a psychiatric history, including hospitalizations, a genuine physical complaint may be seen as a reflection of that history. Healthwise, this can be just as dangerous as overlooking the possible psychiatric component.

This is not just theoretical! As a peer advocate—a person with a diagnosis of mental illness working with others in

The Basics

the mental health system—I've heard a number of complaints about just such a thing happening, with the result being a delay in those individuals' receiving the proper medical attention, or actually finding themselves on a psychiatric unit when their acute symptoms were actually medical. It is a definite issue, and it's why many men and women who pursue help for a mental or emotional disorder are concerned about being labeled because of their illness. Labeling—it's fine for Campbell's Cream of Mushroom soup, but not for us.

15. What is the relationship between anxiety and memory?

Many patients cannot consciously remember the trauma(s) that they have suffered. This disconnection between events and memory can apply to an overwhelming trauma experienced in childhood that they could reconstruct only by hearing from their family details of the story that they had consciously forgotten. It might also lead to repression and an inability to remember the regular kind of abuse and/or neglect that they experienced. Clinically, it often seems that one's anxiety serves as a kind of memory of something experienced earlier in life that was overwhelming. Many patients will explain that just as they feel things are going well and turning their way, they experience a panic attack or heightened sense of anxiety. This response appears to be the body's way of remembering that just as things were feeling good—or he or she was feeling really excited—something perceived as bad actually did happen. Freud referred to this phenomenon when he said that hysterics (patients with physical symptoms stemming from anxiety) suffer primarily from reminiscences. In his paper *Repeating, Remembering, and Working Through,*[7] he suggested that we repeat patterns over and again as ways of remembering what happened to us earlier. These ideas harmonize with what we know from modern neuroscience and the work on procedural memory, or memory for common actions that no longer need a conscious thought to correlate with their action. This principle would explain the onset of certain medical symptoms around the onset of an important anniversary reaction.

An apocryphal story from Anna Freud comes to mind. When Ms. Freud ran nurseries in London for displaced children of World War II, a counselor in the nursery worked for three years regularly with a particular little girl, feeding her donuts on Fridays. Several years later, this counselor went to check on her whereabouts. She easily remembered the child and wondered how she was doing and if she remembered her. The girl said that she seemed to remember once getting a donut from her. This story is important because it shows that our conscious memory serves as a screen for many ins and outs of day-to-day life history. Similarly, working closely with the nature of someone's anxiety symptoms can lead to important memories of childhood, which in turn can lead to a relief of symptoms.

In moments of extreme anxiety, total or partial amnesia of the trauma can occur. It seems that both neurologically and psychologically, locking these memories away, or keeping them from ever being stored, serves to protect us from reexperiencing an overwhelming kind of activity.

16. What is the history of anxiety?

As you might imagine, mankind has been anxious as long as mankind has been in existence. The actual word *anxiety* has as its root *angst*, German for fear.

25

The word *panic* stems from the Greek myth of Pan, the god of fertility and the fields who struck intense, irrational fear into the hearts of travelers in desolate areas.[8] Our anxiety system has been intrinsic to our fight-or-flight survival system, using the oldest of nerves (the nose) as a key scout and showing wiring to the evolutionarily oldest parts of the brain. Multiple recorded episodes of anxiety exist, going back to ancient African tribes, the pygmies of Polynesia, or Native American tribes. Historically, common explanations for anxiety included possession of the body by evil spirits, violation of a cultural taboo, or the loss of the soul. Cure has existed for each of these ailments via exorcism (i.e., removal of the evil spirit), shamanism (i.e., using a healer to restore the lost soul by finding it and returning it to the body), or confession of the taboo violation. In the early 20th century, Freud piggybacked his theories on many of these ideas and used the **hypnosis** technique from Jean-Martin Charcot to, in turn, pioneer **psychoanalysis** as a technique and school of thought. Freud's psychoanalysis serves as the basic forerunner of all modern psychotherapy.

Today, theories of anxiety range from neurobiological to sociological to psychological, and in many of our present treatments, the principles used throughout the history of mankind in the treatment of anxiety still apply. For example, any reasonable psychotherapy restores hope, is done by a socially sanctioned healer, involves some theory of mind, and involves a regular long-term relationship between a healer and the patient. These techniques go back to shamans of the caveman and the ancient Greeks' use of theater or

Hypnosis

a form of therapy in which a therapist induces a patient into an enhanced state of relaxation, possibly allowing for deeper memories or feelings to surface.

Psychoanalysis

a form of intensive psychotherapy, usually 4–5 times per week, conducted with the patient lying on the couch, facing away from the analyst.

temples and philosophy as vehicles to provide relief from anxiety. Living in the 21st century, we have benefited enormously from the input of rational science and its scientific method (as well as **psychopharmacology**) as tools; however, many of the techniques that we use to navigate anxiety have been tried and proven to be true over the history of mankind.[9]

Psychopharmacotherapy

the use of medication, prescribed by psychiatrists, to treat mental illness.

The Basics

17. Why is there such a stigma toward mental illness in general and toward anxiety in particular?

People suffering from anxiety often fear they will be stigmatized, as do many with a wide range of mental experiences. Patients commonly feel they are weak for not being better able to manage their anxiety, as if they had conscious control over their anxiety at those overwhelming times. They might also fear that they are alone, and that if anyone knew how unbearable, empty, needy, panicky, frightened, or defective they felt, they would feel even more isolated. Some patients fear an even more threatening situation—exile from their families for admitting they suffer from anxiety, confessing to what is seen in their family system as shameful or to a loss of self-control with the onset of their symptoms. Perhaps they fear they are going crazy and will suffer beyond anxiety—perhaps from a more profound disorder that, for example, a family member already has. Humans feel ashamed of the nature of our distress and fear rejection by loved ones. These feelings, taken together, lead us to keep our symptoms secret and, commonly, to avoid treatment at any cost. The tragedy of this approach lies in distancing ourselves, not only from the healing aspects of relating to others, but from standard effective treatment modalities available today.

If we only knew on the front end how universal feelings of anxiety can be and how anyone honest with himself or herself knows these internal states to some degree, we could feel great relief. Embracing treatment for anxiety can allow people to feel more integrity within themselves. It can also foster the mending of deep family rifts or facilitate the transition out of a dysfunctional family system in a safe way. Symptomatic anxiety symbolizes the mind's difficulty managing a particular, individual mental struggle—a difficulty understood via competent treatment. Anyone who would stigmatize you for your difficulties might be uncomfortable with his own handling of some aspect of your struggle.

Rick's comments:

I would honestly have to say that I have not been stigmatized by others nearly as much as I've stigmatized myself. This does not mean that those of us diagnosed with a mental illness are free from the type of prejudices and misunderstandings in society that other groups have had to overcome. We're not. It's just that self-stigmatization can be the hardest to overcome because it involves so many types of emotions. I'm sure that I'm not alone in having feelings of shame, worthlessness, inadequacy, and regret, all related at least in part to OCD. Not surprisingly, based on what this part of the book says, keeping my symptoms secret and isolating from others have been a large part of my life because of the illness, yet nobody has ever told me I should isolate or keep secrets. This is the stigmatization that I have imposed upon myself. Then again, you just have to look at the headlines in the tabloids to know that self-stigmatization doesn't suffer from lack of company. Words like "psycho" and "schizo" still blare out at us, long past the time that other words of bigotry and such insensitivity have been banished from the newspapers' vocabularies. Self-stigma, though, is still the worst.

18. How is anxiety useful from an evolutionary perspective?

In their book, *Why We Get Sick*, Drs. Randolph Neese and George Williams[10] address the question of anxiety's greater evolutionary purpose. As discussed earlier, the anxiety system serves as a fight-or-flight system, designed for our protection. In an interesting experiment, guppies were placed in a tank with a smallmouth bass behind a glass separating pane. The experimenters categorized the guppies into three different classes based on their confrontation with the big fish: timid (hid), ordinary (swam away), and bold (eyed the bass). When the glass pane separating the groups was removed and sixty hours passed, 40% of the timid group were alive, while only 13% of the normal group and none of the bold group were alive (those not alive were eaten by the smallmouth bass). This is one of many examples that illustrates how anxiety—like a fire alarm designed to save a life once even if causing a hundred false alarms—protects us. From this point of view, it might be that we do not sufficiently fear certain elements of the modern world, such as nuclear radiation or firearms. Common phobias—of leaving home, flying, driving, receiving group attention, or being trapped in a closed space—all stem from situations which, evolutionarily, would have been quite precarious (being eaten if away from the group, falling from a high place, high speed reminiscent of a predator's attack, being punished, or being trapped in a cave).

In another animal model of anxiety, infant monkeys separated from their mothers become acutely anxious and agitated in an attempt to get their mother's attention. This model is useful in terms of thinking about anxiety as a means of protecting us from separation. The anxious monkeys in this example try to soothe themselves as well as to bring themselves back into their mothers' attention. These animal models teach us of anxiety's adaptive purposes.

19. What is the cost of anxiety?

This question demands both financial answers and human answers. Our country spends billions of dollars per year on the treatment of anxiety, which is the most represented and treated of all mental health problems. Over half of these costs come from the medical treatment of medical problems that stem from anxiety! This fact confirms what most of us who have worked in primary care settings know as clinical truth: that much of primary care focuses on the treatment of anxiety and anxiety-related disorders, that one in five patients is on a **benzodiazepine** for anxiety, and that primary care physicians prescribe 80% of the **antidepressant**/antianxiety drugs in this country. Factor in

Benzodiazepine
a type of medication used to treat anxiety.

Antidepressant
a psychiatric medication that is used to treat not only depression, but a wide range of anxiety symptoms as well.

the amount of days lost from work or the relative lack of productivity experienced due to anxiety, or the amount of violence, alcohol abuse, drug abuse, drunk driving and related lost limbs and lives, and the actual cost of anxiety to this country is staggering.[2]

None of the financial costs approximate the human costs of anxiety, which are legion and often experienced over the course of a lifetime. Anxiety has a nasty habit of hanging around for a long time, far overstaying its welcome, and keeping people from seeking the appropriate treatment. Think of anyone you know who has suffered the loss of a child; a rape; childhood sexual, physical, or emotional abuse; any military veteran who has seen active combat duty and witnessed a fellow soldier be blown to shreds; or any child who has witnessed her parents' regularly beating one another. An individual's world might never feel safe again because once these events have taken place, they become forever etched in the banks of emotional and anxious memory. Inasmuch as these events color the ability to be intimate with others, to feel integrity within one's own skin, or to access and actualize the human ability to use freedom of choice, the costs are incalculable.

Notes

1. American Psychiatric Association. (2000). *Diagnostic and statistical manual of mental disorders* (4th ed., text revision). Washington, DC: American Psychiatric Association.

2. Barlow, D.H. (2002). *Anxiety and its disorders.* New York: The Guilford Press.

3. Freud, S. (1959). Inhibitions, symptoms and anxiety (1926 (1925)). In Strachey, J. (Vol. Ed.), *The standard edition of the complete psychological works of Sigmund Freud: Vol. 20* (pp. 77–178). London: The Hogarth Press and the Institute of Psycho-Analysis.

4. Freud, A. (1946). *The ego and the mechanisms of defence.* New York: International Universities Press, Inc.

5. Vaillant, G. (1995). *Adaptation to Life.* Cambridge, MA: Harvard University Press.

6. LeDoux, J. (1996). *The emotional brain: The mysterious underpinnings of emotional life.* New York: Simon & Schuster.

7. Freud, S. (1959). Remembering, Repeating, Working Through. In Strachey, J. (Vol. Ed.), *The standard edition of the complete psychological works of Sigmund Freud: Vol. 12* (pp. 145–156). London: The Hogarth Press and the Institute of Psycho-Analysis.

8. Schmidt, M.D., Leonard J., Warner, B. (2002). *Panic: Origins, insight, and treatment.* Berkeley, CA: North Atlantic Books.

9. Ellenberger, H. (1970). *The discovery of the unconscious: The history and evolution of dynamic psychiatry.* New York: Basic Books.

10. Nesse, G.W. & Williams, G.C. (1994). *Why we get sick: The new science of Darwinian medicine.* New York: Times Books.

The Basics

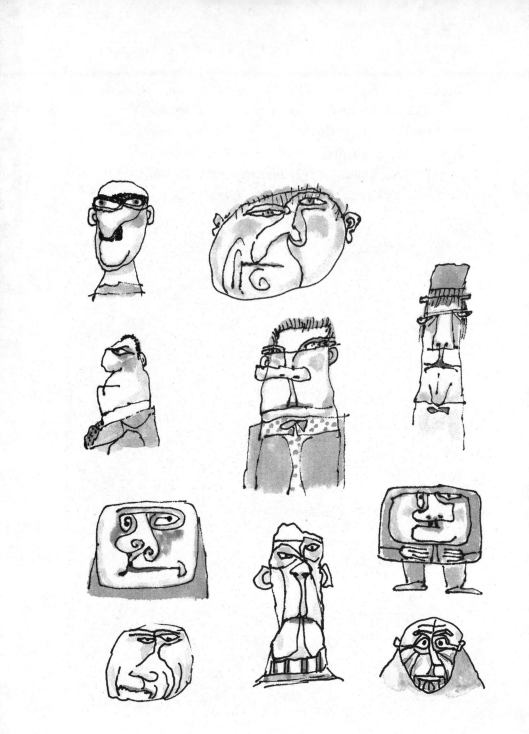

Reprinted with permission from The Cartoon Bank, a division of *The New Yorker* magazine.

PART TWO

The Many Faces of Anxiety

What is performance anxiety?

What causes a panic attack?

Can anxiety really keep me up all night?

More...

20. What is performance anxiety?

We all commonly experience performance anxiety when taking a test, speaking in public, or acting on stage. Patients report all kinds of medical, physical, and psychological symptoms, which range from sweating, nausea, and palpitations to an overwhelming sense of doom to a heightened sense of tension about the potential outcome of their project. This might also happen to accompany an activity which the patient really loves to do (playing her favorite instrument or speaking about the topic which she most enjoys). There often seems to be a history of trauma in these patients. For example, a child made too much noise when practicing a performance and was terrified by the yelling and beating which ensued, thereby feeling threatened by and afraid of his parents. It may take a while working with any particular patient to get to these memories, but it seems that using medication to control the symptoms more immediately while helping the patient to understand that his or her symptoms are not coming out of the blue (as they first seemed), he or she can achieve a greater sense of control. In the case of the child mentioned earlier, this type of understanding provides the now-adult patient with the realization that he does not have to respond to the performance at hand as if it were a time of stern punishment from childhood, when he really did have no control over the overwhelming fear.

Patients also talk about another kind of memory connected to their anxiety surrounding performance: the fear of loss of love from their families. They fear that love in their particular family depends upon performance; hence, a test or other performance becomes not just about delivering the information that they know or communicating the material of the presentation, but rather an assessment of whether they are lovable. This feeling can leave patients feeling angry and hurt that their self-worth has become tied up in a performance rather than simply in a sense of self. In more complicated cases, parents do more than just become critical; they beat their children if the performance is not perfect or beat their children even when the performance is perfect (ostensibly for some trivial item, like the proverbial spilled milk). This unfortunate association places the child in a double bind: damned if he does not succeed, and damned if he does. All of these examples combine the hand that feeds the child intermittently with the one that beats it. This kind of reinforcement—the same principle that keeps people blowing their life savings in Vegas, hoping (in the words of the gambler's prayer) "Lord, let me break even"—keeps children desperately attached to the pursuit of love from an abusive relationship.

Interpretation of success thus becomes complicated. Is a man who recently became the chair of his department competent, powerful, and able to separate from his parents? Or, has he placed himself at risk for a beating? This man might feel proud on the one hand, but become symptomatically anxious on the other as he experiences new-onset rage or panic attacks. It may feel more socially and psychologically acceptable for this man to avoid treatment, live with symptomatic performance anxiety, and keep himself from acting on more aggressive, violent, disruptive feelings.

Rick's comments:

Sometimes at work, but more often in my personal life, I tend to put off activities, even potentially pleasurable ones, because of my anxiety. These undone tasks, which might be minor at first, tend to build up and become more urgent as time passes (such as the bill that comes with a past due notice, or a leaky faucet that goes unfixed). They increase my anxiety over whatever I should have done in the first place. Then the task suddenly looms large and threatening. I'll bet I'm not the only anxiety sufferer who goes through this! Does it sound familiar to some of you? I think of this pattern as procrastination; it's deeper than that, however. I tend to be a perfectionist (not, heaven knows, someone who does things perfectly, just someone who thinks I should do things perfectly), and I worry when I begin a task that I won't do it correctly and then will get down on myself. This happens more often with things that are new to me or when I feel the task does not use one of my strengths. As I wrote earlier, when I overcome this and do the task (finally!), I feel a real sense of achievement.

21. *What causes a panic attack?*

To a neutral observer, the idea of choosing to have a panic attack makes no sense. As uncomfortable as panic attacks are, why would anyone choose to suffer in this manner? Learning the ins and outs of patients' choosing to have panic attacks proves to be useful, as it provides the very means to their recovery. Largely their unconscious choice, patients do not realize why they do this to themselves; how can one feel that something which she perceives as overtaking her stems in fact from an unconscious choice of her own making? However, working with patients with anxiety shows over and over again that the timing of a panic attack in an individual's mind correlates invariably with what she is feeling or doing at that point in her life. Many patients report, in time, that they see having panic attacks as a way to confine themselves within a horrible distress. For example, a patient who becomes excited about taking a trip with his fiancée—literally taking off in life, but also leaving his family for the first time—has a panic attack on the airplane, thus keeping himself from the present experience of the joy of the trip (and reconnects to growing up in the abusive home of his alcoholic, rage-filled father). This phenomenon reminds me of the proverb, "a prisoner grows to love his chains." In fact, this notion may account for prisoners' literal reoffense after release from jail; they report not knowing how to handle the freedom of civilian life and functioning better within the confines of what they find familiar. If we anticipate that the other shoe will drop—that we will be blindsided by fate after feeling so good—it makes more sense to choose a panic attack to feel, psychically, more in control of the disaster by creating it. It is preferable to the sneak attack of what our mind anticipates will invariably occur.

22. Can anxiety really keep me up all night?

Insomnia is one of the beasts of anxiety. Sleeplessness leaves one feeling wasted, fatigued, desperate, and hopeless. Restoring someone's ability to sleep can provide immediate, immeasurable relief. The insomnia of anxiety goes beyond counting sheep. Patients ruminate for hours—staying up all night, staring at the ceiling, or reading for hours without sedative effect. Standard methods of sleep hygiene fail, and often patients may resort to walking long distances to contain their anxiety, in effect becoming lost souls wandering the night. Some become anxious about sleep as a way of fearfully remembering traumas that happened at night; others are simply afraid to lose control of the vigilance over their surroundings they maintain while awake. Women who have been victims of sexual harassment or assault,

Insomnia
difficulty with or an inability to sleep at night.

39

anyone who has been robbed, or victims of other violence can speak to the sleepless nights endured for weeks to months afterwards. Acute loss, whether of a relationship, a job, or one's health can trigger profound insomnia. Nightmares from anxiety can turn an otherwise better night of sleep into a wash. For example, someone may report feeling very tired; but once he gets into bed, he cannot sleep. It becomes important to rule out other causes of insomnia, such as major depression, hypomania/mania, and/or substance abuse. Panic about life events keeps people up at night, and this insomnia encourages or causes patients to seek medical attention.

Rick's comments:

Because I am coping with OCD, I have to be very careful when I go to bed to not begin thinking of unresolved events from the day, longer term concerns, or issues from my past (sometimes 20 years past) that disturb or sadden or anger me. I am capable of staying with these thoughts for hours, replaying them again and again; I sometimes find I have let half the night go by without getting a wink of sleep. Even when I have slept, it's not unusual for me to wake up with a thought or a song in my head that seems to take hold and last for hours. (When the song is "Copacabana" by Barry Manilow, my day is pretty well shot!) OCD, of course, does not take the daytime hours off, and I have to be equally careful to try not to ruminate during the day, as best I can.

23. Can anxiety change my dreams?

It often seems that recurrent dreams correlate with one's anxiety; nightmares invariably do. The anxiety dream I see the most involves tidal waves, which can reflect feeling flooded or drowned by emotion. The meaning of the dream can be as individual as the dreamer and his or her associations to it, but common examples of recurrent dreams include being chased by a knife, being raped, or falling from a high place. Conversely, as patients get treatment for their anxiety, their dreams can reshape as well. One might dream of standing on firmer ground or feeling safer or less alone in the world.

24. What is emotional intelligence, and how does that fit with my anxiety?

The work of Daniel Goleman of Harvard University, best known for his book *Emotional Intelligence*, speaks to basic principles of emotional health. He and others view anxiety as one of the body's primary emotions and defines emotional health in part as the healthy management of anxiety. In this view, the healthier we are, the more appropriate is our anxiety to the situation at hand. He refers to Aristotle's ideal of being angry the right amount at the right time towards the right person for the right reason. The man who comes home from work anxious about the day's events and angry at his boss but kicks his dog instead provides a classic example of emotion out of control.[1]

Other examples abound, such as the employee who cannot let go of the agitation he feels toward a coworker for an odd habit or worry he cannot control over his boss's comment that morning. A woman's inability to stop daydreaming about the love she feels for an unavailable client illustrates the poor efficiency of her emotional system. One's anxiety in these situations serves as a useful barometer inasmuch as one overreacts. Patients often report this kind of anxiety as feeling like an archaic dictator, a beast who demands they respond in a particular way to a given situation.

However, this mode no longer fits the present situation. Anyone suffering intensely from this kind of anxiety says that if he could only tailor his anxiety more appropriately, he would feel so much lighter. The more emotionally intelligent we become, the more likely our anxiety will fit the ambient temperature of the present conditions.

Rick's comments:

Emotionally, I am the perfect example of Aristotle's ideal of being angry the right amount at the right time towards the right person for the right reason. (Yeah, right!) Actually, I frequently dredge up, particularly during times of anxiety and stress, old arguments and angers. I think about people who are long out of my life—sometimes even a long-ago school friend or love interest—who have no real meaning to my life today. If I happen to run into a person, generally a family member, about whom I've been replaying old arguments or issues, I never feel angry toward them the way I do during my private thoughts. The present reality and past issues seem, with me at least, to exist in two totally separate spheres. There are times when these thoughts aren't really intruding—I invite them in! For reasons I still need to work on discovering, I intentionally dwell on some of these past hurts and harms when I am not happy with myself or my life. It affords a kind of grim pleasure that I know could not possibly be good for me. I believe this can be overcome when I am ready to let go of this negative thinking.

25. What is self-soothing, and how does it help anxiety?

We all resort to any manner of behaviors to deal with our anxiety. Generally speaking, these behaviors might be referred to as self-soothing. Some self-soothing behaviors serve more strategically than others. Some patients will choose to exercise, cook a good meal, meditate, take a warm bath, get a good night's sleep, or contact an old friend to comfort themselves when anxious. Others will go on a shopping spree, overeat, drink alcohol to excess, masturbate compulsively, or shoplift. These behaviors seem rooted in trying to settle a deeper anxiety. Attempting to understand the particular nature of the anxiety will help to make sense of the choice of self-soothing behavior, thus facilitating the transition to healthier patterns of adaptation. Shopping sprees might help someone feeling cheapened or ugly to feel worthy and glamorous; binge eating can lead to feeling less empty or more fed by a provider from childhood; drinking may provide a temporary reunification with an old love; masturbation may stave off feelings of abandonment or smallness; and shoplifting may be an attempt to seek the punishment and humiliation one feels he deserves for wanting so much and feeling so greedy.

Rick's comments:

Both the productive and self-destructive things I do to self-soothe work to decrease my anxiety, at least in the short run. The difference is that when I do something positive, such as involving myself in a worthwhile activity, the anxiety stays lowered. When I do something harmful to myself, such as binge eating, the effect lasts only as long as the activity does, and then I find myself more anxious than ever. I know that recovering alcoholics say that when you have a problem and drink over it, you then have one more problem. My drug of choice is food, and I can attest that the results are pretty much the same as for the alcoholic: a problem plus one! The term that I use for the less fortunate choices I make to decrease anxiety is "self-medicating," but self-soothing also describes it pretty well. I like the fact that self-soothing can also apply to my positive ways of warding off anxiety and I'm going to add it to my vocabulary.

26. How are guilt and shame part of anxiety?

Shame

a feeling that accompanies the uncovering of humiliating or embarrassing thoughts or behaviors.

Guilt

a feeling that one has done something wrong.

Superego

also known as the "conscience," one of three theoretical parts of the mind, first established by Sigmund Freud, that represents a person's internal moral compass.

Shame and/or **guilt** go hand in hand with anxiety. These emotions are old, primitive lodestars in our development. It is commonly thought that guilt serves as a more evolved feeling than shame. Guilt has to do with feeling one has broken a particular law or rule and merits punishment. Freud thought that feelings of guilt experienced in childhood became the **superego**, or censor/dictator of the mind that keeps us from acting on our base desires. He also believed that this superego allowed for human civilization to continue. He who feels guilty often seeks a medium for confession in which he can relieve himself of the anxiety over his perceived guilt. The anxiety of guilt is expected; one knew better, especially if he had the poor luck to be caught in the act. Conscious guilt does not rock a sense of self in the same way as shame. One might even joke about it being easier to ask for forgiveness than permission. Unconscious guilt—a feeling that we need to suffer for our actions, and particularly for our successes because we do not deserve them—can wreak havoc on lives as people set themselves up for punishment and then worry (realistically) about the potential consequences of their lying, stealing, cheating, etc. Shame seems to go much deeper. A more primitive emotion, shame represents a deep sense of humiliation, mortification, or defectiveness. We try to hide that of which we are most ashamed. Therefore, patients feeling guilty use treatment to confess that of which they wish to unburden themselves. Those feeling shame tend to keep their anxiety more secret. The roots of this wish to conceal seemingly shameful thoughts and feelings then proves central to their psychotherapy, as undoing these mental constraints offers liberation from a symptom's burden.

Anxious, guilty, shameful feelings often draw from material either sexual or aggressive in nature. Experiencing sexual urges or fantasies which seem socially unacceptable leave us feeling guilty, unsafe, or ashamed. Likewise, feeling hostile, aggressive yearnings can seem intolerable. The anxiety over having these wishes yet not feeling comfortable having them—let alone talking about them—prompts our minds to handle or not handle this dilemma. For instance, a patient who begins to wash his hands compulsively may report that he feels dirty for pursuing a woman exclusively for her vagina; he washes out of a perceived need for punishment. A woman who presents to the emergency room with an acute sense of chest pain from a panic attack may coincidentally report in a careful history that she has started an extramarital affair. A boy who becomes sexually involved with a male relative at a young age may develop compulsive symptoms to be sure. He may in addition feel the need to hide his sexual secret for fear of being discovered, not only for having such deep sexual longings but also for having ones that involve a male.

Rick's comments:

If my baseball skills had been honed as sharply as my sense of guilt and shame, I might be playing third base for the Yankees! I think a lot of my anxiety—my OCD—has to do with control. I use both my thoughts and rituals to maintain or to try to maintain a sense of control. At the same time, I feel controlled by the rituals, thoughts, and behaviors

I act out on. This need for control is, I'm sure, based on guilt and shame, and the nature of my OCD is such that I relive the guilty feelings and what has led to them again and again. When these feelings have a hold of me, they become the entire focus of how I see myself; and this causes shame.

What have I pronounced myself guilty of? Spending a lot of my adult life as a recluse or feeling unworthy of being with people are common accusations. For example, at one point in my life, I would make plans to be with friends and then always get sick and be unable to join them. Eventually this pattern cost me all my friends. Also, I left law school in my first year and did not return. The fallout from these actions—like not starting a family, or being under- or unemployed for years—has caused me shame and, ironically, has intensified the feelings and behaviors that caused the problems in the first place. I don't know how or why or what purpose it serves, but I'm pretty sure that my biological mom's illness and death when I was very young are behind a lot of my guilt and, therefore, my OCD and anxiety. That's a shame, given the fact that my mom loved me and would only want the best for me. Is this all a vicious cycle? Yup. Has it made me feel hopeless or like giving up? Nope.

27. How can my culture shape the way I experience anxiety?

Culture plays a role in the presentation of one's anxious symptoms in the same way that an organism always responds to its particular niche. The creation of a common, socially accepted medium through which anxiety can present itself has become a recognized part of cultural history for millennia, always being a part of the written records. One way to think of this dynamic involves the concept of a symptom pool, i.e., that any given culture has its own various symptoms which it sanctions as permissible outlets for the experience anxiety. In Haiti or other cultures bound by voodoo, someone experiencing anxiety may be seen as under the spell of a root. In Puerto Rico, the syndrome *ataque de nervios* is well known; in Asian cultures, *Amok* (a period of withdrawn brooding followed by violent outbursts, all of which is denied and forgotten later) and *Koro* (a fear of genital retraction, often after sexual involvement) are well known. A woman experiencing anxiety in the United States today may choose the outlet of an eating disorder from amongst the available symptoms in the pool. In caricature, every New Yorker becomes neurotic and ends up on a psychoanalyst's couch. Or, different cultures may vary in their sanctioning versus prohibiting the use of alcohol or marijuana.

Culture also affects anxiety manifestations in their stigmatization. In either Indian or Asian cultures, for example, members can feel that suffering from anxiety indicates weakness. Often, families guard generations of secrecy and shame surrounding a family history of mental illness. The institutionalization, suicide attempts, domestic violence, or drug addiction of any family member can lead to stigmatization regardless of culture. Fear of showing weakness leads to continuation of the conspiracy of silence. As family members continue to torture themselves with their own anxiety symptoms and remain in isolation, children and young adults suffering from anxiety can grow up to become the same restricted parents they swore they would never become.

Finally, culture can allow for differing philosophical structures. In the West, we have tended to see the mind as separate from the body for more than 500 years; we are only now starting to look meaningfully at the impossibility of separating mind from body. We like to see problems as relating to their **pathophysiology**; we like to prove ideas with studies that sustain rigorous statistical analysis, often pooling large samples of data together. In the East, mind and body never parted company. The life force chi defines health; doctors receive a salary until a patient becomes ill; and traditional healing methods only now undergoing rigorous scientific methodological testing coexist naturally with Western techniques. Asian cultures allow for the power of the mind to profoundly shape a size of one human life.

Pathophysiology
the mechanisms of disease processes in the body and the ways in which disease alters normal structure and function.

28. How does anxiety affect my personality?

In seeing anxiety as a disorder (e.g., "he has panic attacks" or "he suffers from obsessive-compulsive disorder"), we miss other ways in which anxiety can shape a personality. This type of anxiety becomes more of a stance we take to survive. For example, a man who seems self-centered and entitled (narcissistic) becomes anxious when attention shifts away from himself; therefore, he strategically places himself in the center of action. He may boast, fail to relate or listen to others, or listen but be mainly interested in how he may use others for his own advancement, all to confirm his own special nature. In so doing, he alleviates his own anxiety of fearing abandonment or feeling small and unimportant. Those acutely anxious about separation (sometimes called borderline) fear being alone. Couples may often find that they fight the night before one is to leave the other, with one of the couple threatening to hurt himself or herself in response to being left. This hijacking behavior keeps couples deeply connected, thus avoiding the feared abandonment. A thief may steal to avoid feeling deep tides of unworthiness. This anxiety characterizes shoplifters who steal items of trivial monetary value, demonstrating to themselves that they feel deserving of these objects. A more flamboyant, attention-seeking (otherwise known as histrionic) character may deeply fear being forgotten, which translates to feeling unloved. Her large displays of unforgettable behavior leave her always remembered, if not endeared. An obsessive-compulsive person may feel dirty or bad and may engage in highly calculated behavior to undo these feelings. Washing her hands alleviates the dirty feeling; constantly checking the stove or the lock can undo her feelings of explosive rage. Those who avoid social situations may, in their hearts, assume their perceived inevitable rejection ahead of time and thus avoid public events.

29. What if I fear inadequacy?

Classically known as Alfred Adler's term, "inferiority complex," the fear of inadequacy characterizes much of human behavior and much of anxiety. Common manifestations of this fear include feeling short, childish, insufficient, not fully a man, not fully a woman, or defective in some basic way. Fear of inadequacy does not equal inadequacy, as some of the most gifted, successful people remain driven by this underlying fear. These perceptions of the self as inadequate can stem from family histories where parents cause a child to feel that he or she is only as lovable as his or her performance. The child's mind may then equate performance with love. Because it is impossible for anyone to perform perfectly, anything can potentially feel inadequate. Other feelings of defectiveness can arise from actual defects, which we all have. We are all born with our flaws, some more externally visible than others— be they a birth defect, a childhood history of medical illness, a learning disability, a stammer, a history of bed-wetting, or a naturally quick temper. Criticism of these flaws can be very hurtful, as we all know that the criticisms that are the most true, or that we feel to be the most true, are the most difficult to hear. Avoiding these hurtful feelings and their accompanying anxiety is only natural.

External compensatory behaviors help some of us to try to fill the gap. Sometimes, they are disturbing. Hate crimes including, but not limited to, homophobic violence, racism, or sexual harassment stem from a profound sense of inadequacy on the part of the perpetrator. In picking a victim whom he perceives to be weaker, he attempts to dominate in order to feel superior. Social situations can elicit less severe types of compensation. A man may attend a party and see someone he has had a crush on but who has rejected him before. He might continue to maintain his romantic interest in this person but still fear absolute rejection. Perhaps that fear feels like an uncontrollable anger that radiates from his gut and spirals out of control. These feelings of rejection might overlap with the very feeling of powerlessness experienced in his childhood, when an actual lack of protection or rejection by his family (people whom he so badly wanted to be close to) did occur. This pain might trigger the compensation of drug or alcohol use, in an attempt to look for feelings of power and attractiveness.

30. What is the role of stress and its contribution to anxiety?

We know from laboratory research with rats and from common sense that external stress leads to anxiety. Stress comes in many types, including but not limited to overwork, inadequate sleep, single parenting, two-career marriages, transition from one culture to another, change of job, divorce, death of a loved one, sickness in a loved one, or living with a medical or mental illness. Stress lowers the barrier of any potential event to make someone anxious; physiologically, stress, as the body sees it, is anxiety in overdrive. Dr. Bruce McEwen of Rockefeller University has studied the long-term impact of stress and concluded that in chronic stress, the very chemical changes that help us fight or flee can create damage over the long run. Hence, we find immune system weakness, heart damage, damaged memory capacity, change in fat deposits, bone demineralization, and chronic anxiety or aggression in lieu of increased alertness and readiness to run or fight. These kinds of thoughts are the backbone of the new field called **psychoneuroimmunology**, which has directly linked the stress we experience with a decrease in immune function or increased disposition to get sick or perhaps develop cancer. These studies help clarify the inseparability of the mind from the body.

Psychoneur-immunology
the study of the ways in which the neurological immunological mental systems interface (for example, getting a cold during times of high stress).

31. What is separation anxiety?

It seems that much of anxiety stems from a basic fear of being alone or being left by those close to us. This separation anxiety starts in childhood, as the child separates from his/her mother and learns to navigate the world. A child who ventures out from his mother to return safely and receive a warm welcome back learns to feel that separation can be safe. If the child's leaving the mother threatens the mother, however, a different response ensues. A mother may have lost a prior child from an accident, naturally making her more wary. Perhaps she feels so dependent and needy herself that the child's leaving rattles her sense of security (e.g., women who have children to stave off their own loneliness). Children of such mothers may receive a yell or spank in response to their adventures or as a function of their caretaker's agitation. The theory is that these children learn that leaving can create a particular kind of anxiety in their caretaker and learn not to leave as a way to protect themselves and their caretakers.

These reactions to separation are far preferable to early abandonment by the mother. We know from human life and monkey experiments that early neglect leads to permanent nerve, brain, and personality damage. Rat pups separated from their mothers at birth but then reunited after a while have much higher levels of stress; monkeys fed by a mechanical mother become permanently brain damaged; and the babies from the Romanian orphanages who have chronic difficulties with **attachment** serve as testimony to the critical nature of early maternal stimulation and closeness.

Attachment

the process of bonding to another human being during the course of development.

Separation shows up in many adult symptoms. Patients can experience their first bouts of anxiety, depression, eating disorders, or drug abuse as they leave home for college, literally becoming homesick. Two partners about to separate from one another for a temporary but extended period of time fight as a way to deeply connect with one another before the separation. They also confirm that the other partner is of no value, making it is easier to say goodbye than if the partner were truly esteemed. In therapy, separation from the therapist can become a major parameter of examination, as patients often develop strong reactions, old feeling states (e.g., sadness or feelings of inadequacy), or relapses of symptoms (e.g., relapses into drug abuse or sexual promiscuity) before a separation from the therapist.

Rick's comments:

The first major loss in my life resulted from the illness and death of my biological mom when I was 8 (my father later remarried and I am fortunate to have a wonderful step-mom). For years, Mom suffered from multiple sclerosis, and we were often separated due to her hospitalizations. The most noticeable result of the anxiety I was feeling during that time was my going from being a skinny kid to an overweight kid. My binge eating patterns—that have never totally ended—began at that time. This was my first bout with depression and, I believe, OCD. Binge eating, whether being done by an 8-year-old in 1962 or a 48-year-old in 2002, doesn't have much to do with hunger; it's emotional eating, a warding off of anxiety, and it can stick around long after the reasons for that anxiety have ended. It's why, when I'm struggling with food issues, I can still sometimes feel like an 8-year-old.

32. How are sadism and masochism connected to anxiety?

Sadism and **masochism** are commonly misunderstood to involve uniquely sexual behaviors. However, in their more everyday presentations, they help us to understand profound separation anxiety. Sadism and

Sadism
a style of thinking and behavior that involves a desire, either conscious or unconscious, to punish or to be dominant over others.

Masochism
a style of thinking and behavior that involves a desire, either conscious or unconscious, to be punished or to be submissive to another.

53

masochism house different sides of the same coin. The golden rule of sadomasochism is to do unto others what was once done to oneself in one's past. Sexual behaviors of sadism and masochism are extensions of the psychological principles that follow.

A sadist (a term that comes from the Marquis de Sade) does unto others. A child will choose abuse over neglect any day of the week; children growing up in abusive homes learn that abuse is one way of relating deeply to their caretakers. Patterns of domestic violence illustrate this phenomenon. A violent husband may fear rejection from his wife because she has been promoted at work and thus will be less available to tend to him. He fears that she will leave him. When he perceives this threat, he responds by becoming violent toward her. Thus, he recreates the closeness he felt when his own father beat him. In this way he feels less afraid of being left. Often, he may even prompt his wife, the victim, to leave temporarily in order to bring back to life the feelings of loneliness and worthlessness he most feared to begin with and which led to the violent behavior. Once the cycle has completed, it can repeat all over, a pattern which reinforces the behavior more deeply.

A masochist (a term from Leopold von Sacher-Masoch) develops an internal relationship in which he does to himself that which was done to him. Therefore, he never has to separate from his caretakers. A common example of masochism would be self-deprecation. The masochist feels overwhelmed with anxiety of abandonment, fearing being left for his sense of hatefulness or worthlessness. This psychological pain can become so unbearable that he will either directly abuse himself or find someone to do so. Self-abuse can include viewing oneself harshly, binging on food, abusing drugs, creating trouble with the law, or seeking promiscuous, risky sex. Masochists recreate the abusive situations that they experienced, thus becoming like the parents who were abusive towards them. This method shifts them out of their own pain by allowing them to feel more like their parents (and therefore closer). Giving oneself this kind of a beating proves (in the masochist's mind) that he or she is more valuable than the feeling of nothingness, which can be his or her deepest fear. Placing so much focus on the pain of a beating can also attempt, in a kind of self-regulatory mechanism, to keep those deeper overwhelming feelings (e.g., abandonment, nothingness, or feelings of disintegration) from spilling out of control.

33. What if I self-mutilate to manage my anxiety?

Examples of **self-mutilation** are common extensions of masochism. You may have purposely cut or burned yourself; you may have purposely scarred your hands, wrists, arms, or legs as a result of self-mutilation. The movie *The Piano Teacher* illustrates perfectly this behavior and its psychology. Self-mutilation serves to manage overwhelming anxiety. Usually, patients report that physical pain feels much more bearable than the psychic pain that they are experiencing at the time. The psychic pain may stem from violent urges towards significant others, or from otherwise intolerable feelings of annihilation, disintegration, or the like. Redirecting the violence toward oneself contains these urges and thus prevents one from hurting people whom one also genuinely feels that one needs. Self-mutilation serves as a compromise between expressing the violence and containing it in a way that will not hurt others. This self-punishment can often feel soothing, as the mutilation serves to take the greater psychic pain away. It also

Self-mutilation
the practice of injuring oneself, usually by cutting, burning, or piercing.

55

recreates a union with the abusive parent who related to the child abusively, thus helping the patient to feel less alone, annihilated, or disintegrated.

In a less overt way, people mutilate themselves figuratively with their harsh internalized voices. Telling oneself how inadequate and horrible and nonsensical one is serves a similar purpose—keeping the pain in check, but also redirecting the rage towards oneself to protect the caretaker. These beatings can make self-mutilators feel very powerful, a genuine contrast to the sense of helplessness experienced otherwise (either from separation or another type of annihilation).

34. Is body modification a sign of anxiety?

Tattoos and piercings have become fixtures of American culture. Various cultures across the world have used body modification for centuries. The roots of this behavior, culturally as well as psychologically, are deep. But most people with a tattoo will tell you that they have chosen this brand of art as a way to make note of something important. It seems that the meaning of the particular tattoo can be as individual as the person who chose it or the circumstances under which she decided to have it done. I believe the relative permanence of this style of art can reflect an underlying separation anxiety. A man who feels insecure and small may choose to bond with the permanent image of a naked woman on his skin, thus feeling strong and manly when displaying this image to his friends. This image and his view of himself with this image help reduce his underlying anxiety of feeling small and childlike. It might also keep his friends' eyes on him, giving him a kind of attention that leaves him feeling less alone or abandoned.

Piercings involve similar logic. They relay to the recipient an external confirmation of being special but do so in a self-mutilatory way. A girl may pierce her tongue to announce that she is sexually potent, yet, in doing so, she also permanently reminds herself that she feels her mouth is dirty and (in her perception) in need of punishment for these sexual wishes. As with tattoos, only the wearer can genuinely convey either the particular meaning of any piercing or any potential anxiety that wearing it might alleviate.

35. What if I am so lonely I feel I could die?

Loneliness can create overwhelming anxiety, and anxiety can reinforce loneliness. Ultimately we are on our own in life, and much of the perceived emptiness we can feel when alone can drive our struggle to be relevant in life or, perhaps, to deny that we will die alone. Its extreme form is the avoidant personality, a person who wishes deeply to be connected to the world around him but just as deeply fears rejection. Another common loneliness is that of depression, where a feeling of not being lovable can breed a toxic isolation. This brand of loneliness further reinforces feelings of inadequacy, thus reinforcing the isolation.

We can also feel emotionally lonely despite physical connection with someone. A couple may be together in a relationship but the individuals might still experience profound anxiety and yearnings to feel more understood and less lonely. Loneliness can range from simple sadness to a kind of empty, desperate, soul-searching, frenetic feeling to a deep sense of worthlessness. This loneliness can prompt impulsive, desperate maneuvers to manage one's internal state. Filling one's self with illegal substances, sex, food, people, or material goods can reflect panic over one's sense of emptiness, thus illustrating the basic connection between internal loneliness and manipulation of the external environment. Treatment of anxiety can help you to feel less alone with your anxiety; to restructure your internal world so that you can feel more comfortable being alone; to appeal less to the outside world as a way of regulating these feelings of loneliness; and to accept this loneliness as you go through it as a fundamental condition of humanity.

Rick's comments:

While I have been fortunate enough through my work to be much less alone than I used to be, my most powerful urge is still to isolate. A weekend spent by myself, which by Sunday night has me feeling depressed and useless, doesn't seem to prevent my arranging things so that I'm just as alone the following weekend. Part of it is my refusal to overeat when others are around. The wiser voice in my head whispers "Good! So be around other people and don't overeat—kill two birds with one stone." Who can heed that voice, though, when another one is shouting "Good! So let go of other people and dig in!" The fact that I still listen to that voice so often is not a source of pride to me.

Another part is self-consciousness. Because of my OCD and the sense of being an outsider it causes, of not being one of the—to use a great phrase by the late, great advocate known as Howie the Harp—"chronically normal," I know it's not unusual for anybody to think at times "if they only knew the real me." The anxiety, however, definitely makes that feeling more intense.

36. Is my rage related to anxiety?

Aggression is one of the most common responses to anxiety. Bar fights, stalking behaviors, sexual violence, road rage, or abuse of prisoners all come to mind. Aggression is the fight part of the fight-or-flight response. In a deeper way, aggression helps protect us from a feared threat. Aggression helps us to act powerfully against the fear experienced inside; the aggressor goes from feeling passive and helpless to active and strong, even though in reality he may become out of control. He also becomes connected to his victim, an important factor if the underlying threat is abandonment. In attempting to understand aggression, it becomes useful to examine what the threat might be in any given situation. Bar fights may result from the perception that a man's wife or girlfriend is being stolen. Sexual violence can be caused by feeling too feminine and wanting to undo the discomfort by making someone else feel humiliation; abusing prisoners of war can stem from one's own anxiety of annihilation in wartime.

37. What if I am anxious that my spouse is cheating on me?

At times, patients report concern over their spouse's fidelity. Actually verifying that the spouse is or is not cheating can prove helpful, as spouses can feel anxious for years only to learn that for several years, in fact, their spouse has cheated. Wanting to deny news of this magnitude, even if it happens under one's nose, occurs frequently. Long absences from a spouse, not allowing or not welcoming a spouse to accompany one on business trips, or a sudden change in sexual wishes in the context of a long-standing pattern of sexual relations with a spouse can all indicate possible infidelity.

More commonly, one's spouse is not cheating and the fear that he or she is cheating represents a deeper fear of being left and a lack of trust. Becoming excited about being together in a relationship can precipitate fearing the worst. A woman whose father left her at a young age—either by divorcing his wife for a woman with whom he was having an affair or dying—may re-experience this fear of loss in her present romantic relationship. Fearing infidelity recreates the feeling of loss and devaluation; it can carry a sense of internal blame. Thus, the woman might feel responsible for her husband's imagined infidelity, blaming herself for some perceived inadequacy such as no longer feeling sexy enough nor publicly charming enough. This self-blame might spare her partner her own rage, which may reflect a stockpile of the same feelings of rage and worthlessness that the she felt as a girl when her father left or died. Fearing this infidelity and the low self-worth that accompanies the fantasy reunites the woman with a familiar feeling of being left. Inasmuch as this feeling is familiar, it decreases her anxiety about new kinds of trust or happiness which could occur in her intimate relationship.

38. Does pregnancy cause anxiety?

Pregnant women and their partners or couples wishing to conceive can experience several phases of anxiety. The first is that of contemplating pregnancy. Potential parents wonder if they are ready for the responsibilities ahead, also wondering if it might be easier to avoid that responsibility. Others might feel calmed by the prospect, as they might feel the role of a parent will be easier than that of a spouse. Perhaps this notion stems from an underlying fear of separation, as the parent contemplating pregnancy knows that a child cannot abandon him or her in the same way that a spouse can.

A second phase of this anxiety comes with the actual pregnancy. It becomes important for the therapist and the anxious parents to understand whether the child is wanted and planned. If so, despite the happiness and joy the potential child may bring, a woman may struggle with her own fears of actually becoming a mother, as can a man about becoming a father. If the baby was not wanted, the couple may feel a different kind of anxiety—whether to continue the pregnancy. These decisions are never easy. Even if a woman believes in her heart that it is the right thing to terminate the pregnancy, feelings about an abortion can surface in all kinds of ways over the years, perhaps in wondering what would have happened had she carried the child to term. These feelings become particularly heightened if delaying the onset of parenthood means dealing with infertility issues later in the union. It seems that the human psychology does not respond as concretely to abortion as can the legislature, with the man and/or woman unconsciously feeling that they have murdered a child. If the potential mother and father are not together in a steady relationship, many more anxieties rise to the surface, involving the fate of the child, decisions about the relationship's course, questions of child support and custody, cultural and family expectations of the woman, and the like. Regardless of outcome, these decisions do not come without profound emotional anxieties.

Finally, as the continued pregnancy develops, multiple changes occur in the woman's body, which may lead to overt anxiety. Nausea of morning sickness is uncomfortable, and women are also anxious to know how long it will last. The anxiety of having one's body change so drastically in ways involving a loss of control (weight, urine output, bowel functions) can trigger questions of security. All the while, expectant parents always wonder if the baby will be healthy and how they will cope with their new parental responsibilities.

39. Can anxiety affect my or my spouse's ability to get pregnant?

Regrettably, some doctors deliver bad news badly. This delivery can occur in obstetric infertility clinics as much as in any other specialty. Telling a woman that she is sterile or a man that he has a low sperm count can be devastating, especially since a couple that has not been able to conceive often wants a child more than they have ever wanted anything in their lives. Sometimes this diagnosis is accurate, and sometimes it is not. Most of us know of cases where a couple tries and tries unsuccessfully to have a child. After giving up hope and beginning the adoption process, they conceive successfully. At least one factor contributing to this phenomenon is a relaxation of anxiety. Once a couple stops trying to conceive, their attention goes elsewhere, even if to the grieving process. This distraction may allow the body to relax enough (and lower the stress hormone cortisol, which impacts the brain's secretion of the female hormones needed for pregnancy) to allow pregnancy, much as an athlete can perform better if attention is, in part, directed away from the performance at hand. The work of Alice Domar at Harvard's Mind/Body Center for Women's Health suggests that letting go of the focus to have a baby and using relaxation and guided visual imagery to relax—focusing on personal happiness—can do wonders to treat anxiety. Paradoxically, 44% of women with infertility in her study became pregnant. The point is not to offer false hope, but to illustrate that the stress of anxiety at a molecular level is real and can have a direct impact on your health and fertility. Getting treatment for your anxiety can improve your life, whether you have a child or not.

40. What is sexual anxiety?

Not surprisingly, sexual relations are a common medium through which people experience and express anxiety. Avoidance of sexual activity is one of the most common manifestations of sexual anxiety. Patients who do so may have a particular phobia of sexual intercourse and try to keep themselves safe from dangers they imagine will occur in a sexual situation. Sexual intercourse in general, and orgasm in particular, involve a loss of bodily control. Fears of overwhelming excitement or of fusion with a lover may lead to fantasies of lost control and destruction. In French, the nickname for orgasm is *le petit mort* (the small death).

Another sexual anxiety is a fear of intense sexual gratification or sexual success. A patient might begin a happy sexual relationship. As the partners become more emotionally close, they may start to imagine their worlds imploding. This anxiety can take the form of fear of contracting a sexually transmitted disease, unwanted pregnancy with their partner (despite using standard methods of birth control), or feelings of newly discovered defectiveness in the partner. This sexual anxiety can often be understood in the context of one's family history. It is not uncommon for people who grow up in homes where sex and sexuality were not spoken about directly to fear intercourse. A child who grows up without a role model for the comfortable handling of sexual desire and behavior is left alone to figure out how to navigate this new experience. Thus the joy of sex can feel something like getting in over one's head. A child with a history of sexual abuse or with a parental history of sexual abuse can seldom engage in sexual experiences without some degree of wariness, at least on an unconscious anxiety level. Or, someone deeply attached in his or her relationship with a parent (daughter-mother, son-mother, daughter-father, son-father) can associate sexual activity with one's partner as permanently leaving one's parents. Feelings of sexual joy can feel illegal, dangerous, and liberating, thereby causing partners to create all manner of havoc for themselves in their minds as they relate sexually.

Some sexual anxiety presents symptomatically as an inability to perform. Women can experience vaginismus (or clamping of the vaginal musculature, thus preventing entry of the penis). Other women experience anorgasmia, or the inability to achieve orgasm. Likewise, men may be unable to sustain an erection, may maintain an erection but be unable to ejaculate, or may ejaculate prematurely. These anxieties about intimate human relationships involving loss of control become magnified when sexual activity begins. With a skilled professional, these interpersonal struggles and/or sexual anxieties can be treated with success.

41. What if I am anxious that I might be gay?

Another sexual anxiety is homosexual anxiety. Discussing sexuality in general, or homosexuality and bisexuality in particular, can make people uncomfortable, if not frankly anxious. With a drive as strong as human sexuality—a force which draws on our biology, objects of desire, fantasies, behavior with others, our family/social/religious morals, and, possibly, our histories of abuse—it makes sense that people react strongly to views that differ from their own. Because homosexual notions, feelings, behaviors, and histories have the capacity to evoke such complex anxieties, it makes sense to understand them more closely. Simply reviewing Freud's basic tenet that we are all born with an inherent bisexuality (based on an infant's love for his or her mother and father) can help to reassure any person struggling with a homosexual type of anxiety. An open-minded attitude can allow for conversations in which these anxieties can be worked through to unfold. Several common examples follow.

It is not uncommon for a heterosexual person to believe that he or she may be homosexual because he or she finds other people of the same gender to be physically attractive. This anxiety can snowball into deep concern; patients may even seek treatment in the emergency room late at night wondering if they are gay (known as homosexual panic). In many instances, it seems that this homosexual anxiety actually prevents people from pursuing heterosexual relationships. In this seeming contradiction, a heterosexual who intensely desires the opposite sex—but fears emotional and/or sexual intimacy at the same time—may prefer to fear being gay. This stance keeps him or her from acting on his or her feared heterosexual desires. These homosexual attractions can thus hijack a man's ability to be with a woman, or a woman's ability to be with a man. In these instances, homosexual anxiety serves as a disguise for heterosexual anxiety.

Another common homosexual anxiety stems from longings for one's absent mother, father, or other significant caretaker. A man who grew up with no father, or with a father who was physically present but emotionally removed, may consciously remember so painfully wishing that his father would pay attention to him. He may long for all that did not happen with his father, be it trips, sports, or simply regular emotional involvement. Though this man may feel as heterosexual as the next in his conscious desires and masturbation fantasies, he may find himself longing for deep intimacy with a man. He may then find himself fearing he is gay because these yearnings leave him anxious and without the tools a male role model might have taught him about handling these feelings. He may respond to these fears with compulsive heterosexual activity (the so-called Don Juan complex) to reassure himself that he is not gay; he may find himself experimenting with homosexual activity to test these desires; or he may find himself drinking excessively with men at bars or parties in male-bonding activities. The anxiety of being around and with men in more intimate settings may feel homosexual in nature, prompting him to use alcohol to treat his anxiety and thus attempt to bury these longings which feel so dangerous and forbidden. The same could occur reciprocally for a woman with her mother.

Other times the real issue is allowing oneself to come out—to acknowledge publicly what one knows and may have known for many years to be true about oneself: that one is gay. In my clinical experience, it seems that male homosexuality declares itself earlier and more firmly than female homosexuality. I have seen many more lesbian women who could imagine being with a man and raising a family than I have seen gay men contemplating the reciprocal situation. Gay men and women commonly raise families with their same-sex partners. In these instances, the issue becomes allowing one to accept one's true self. With devastating results, the psychiatric community for years diagnosed homosexuality as a disease and attempted to correct the "illness" by providing reparative therapy. Homosexual anxiety responds to no longer feeling compelled to deny an aspect of one's nature, a process which would be a part of any good psychotherapy.

42. What if I am nervous about what I am going to do with my life?

This question provokes waves of anxiety, not just in individuals but in their families and cultures. As humans, we all ask what we are meant to do with our lives, and when doing it, we ask how it matches with what we think we want. People who love their work invariably feel better and happier than those who do not. What keeps people from finding work they love becomes an interesting question; will they find a reason not to enjoy any work as a function of their personality, or will a change of career offer that which was always missing?

The Many Faces of Anxiety

67

Patients who have loved working and can no longer do so report a mourning process, like with any other death. Patients who work seem universally happier than those who do not, and those who work in settings which maximize their native gifts seem to thrive even more. Patients who have become unemployed panic not only about what to do but about how to stay afloat financially. Those that work but hate their jobs might wonder about the nature of their true callings.

Help is available. If you struggle to know what your true calling might be, there are basic steps which do not involve epiphanies. You can test yourself for career change (vocational testing); you can seek career counseling; or you can read about people who have struggled with these questions and found ways through the anxiety. I recommend starting with Po Bronson's *What Should I Do With My Life?*[2] If these basic steps do not yield the results you are looking for, you may be an ideal candidate for psychodynamic psychotherapy (see Treatment Section).

43. What is the role of perfectionism and procrastination in anxiety?

If we experience a fear of inadequacy, we fear that our efforts will be viewed as imperfect. These fears speak to our wish to perform ideally. In an extreme form, we become perfectionistic and obsessive-compulsive. The wish to be flawless can be so powerful that, paradoxically, it leads us to procrastinate. The stalling allows us to imagine that we could create the perfect project (an impossibility) when we start; therefore, when our project meets criticism, it becomes instead a function of not having enough time. We trick ourselves into thinking that if we only had more time, it could be ideal.

Procrastination, in turn, can lead to a withholding personality style. We delay the delivery of a project with the idea that we will do it perfectly at some point. In the meanwhile, we delay delivery of the material in a passively sadistic style to the person who wants it. This pattern attempts to make the intended recipient suffer (feel withheld from love and praise), much as we felt when we felt so devalued or imperfect when receiving criticism for our earlier efforts.

Rick's comments:

I identify very strongly with the idea that a need to be perfect, or to do something perfectly, can lead to procrastination. When I make mistakes, even minor ones, it seems to go right to the core of my sense of self, validating every negative thought I have about who I am. My pattern is to be repetitious, both in what I do and in what I avoid doing, sticking with the things I have a history of succeeding at, rather than attempting things at which I could (oh, no!) fail, and putting off the things, procrastinating, that I'm not sure I will do well.

I've occasionally heard alcoholics described as "failed perfectionists," and I imagine this term applies to men and women with other types of addictions and to OCDers like me who, having sustained the wound of even a minor mistake or flaw in oneself, can't seem to stop the bleeding.

44. What if I feel totally helpless?

You are not alone, as feeling helpless is such a common feeling in dealing with overwhelming anxiety. It is important to remember that even though you may feel

The Many Faces of Anxiety

helpless, you do not have to continue to feel that way. Making sense of the kind of helplessness you feel can better direct your recovery.

Patients often describe helplessness as a feeling of total misery—a stance of total vulnerability and inability to control the outcome of a given situation. At times referred to as impotent rage, feeling washed ashore by a tidal wave of anxiety, caught in a hurricane of demeaning demons, or grappling with death, the mental experience of helplessness is uncomfortable. Patients will do anything to avoid it, accounting for the phenomenon of agoraphobia, or avoiding any setting in which this feeling might strike again.

Helplessness might take on many meanings. It could be evolutionarily adaptive, much as a farmer might not plant crops in a scorched field or a businessman might not invest in a company that was bankrupt. It might be used as a way to gain the advantage of the sick role in order to obtain love and affection from others. Helplessness might provide the medium in which to express powerful passive aggression, using our own impotent rage to hijack others into feeling helpless. Helplessness might serve in the spirit of beating ourselves, giving us the justification we need to call ourselves defective. This despair might prompt us to resort to drugs and alcohol to feel some power. Other situations in life are so overwhelmingly destructive that feelings of helplessness and despair are completely realistic. In these situations (terrorism on September 11, 2001, for example), there really is nothing that anyone can do to fix a person's pain. We can only try to provide comfort, a listening, safe environment, medication and appropriate therapy as indicated, and to allow for wounds of this kind of helplessness to repair themselves, much as a physical wound scars eventually.

45. What if I fear commitment?

People have anxiety about all kinds of interpersonal commitments. By simple decision theory, saying "yes" to one option means saying "no" to another. Jokes help to alleviate the gravity of this fear in our culture. A man may call himself "commitmently challenged" or "serially monogamous." Marriage may be called a wonderful institution, but who would want to live in an institution? Fear of the interpersonal intensity that goes hand-in-hand with intimacy can make us wary of getting in too deep. Often, these anxieties surface in the context of dating exclusively, cohabitation, engagement, marriage, pregnancy and/or birth of a child, promotion or hire at work, or a medical illness in one of the partners. Any event which potentially intensifies human closeness can ratchet up corresponding fears of commitment. Starting psychotherapy can likewise produce the very fear which people have in their relationships outside of the treatment, thus providing the raw material so helpful to knowing more about this nervousness and providing relief for its pressure.

This anxiety can reflect many different fears. With commitment can come the next phase of developmental life, including raising and providing for a family or starting a business. It can also involve trusting a partner to be emotionally present or trusting in oneself enough to leave one's family of origin. In the most intense way, this anxiety can represent a fear of being annihilated, trapped, or lost in ways yet undiscovered. Being committed means being able to sustain one's own sense of self-worth while simultaneously allowing for and compromising with the values of others. It means allowing for greater flexibility and loss of control than one perceives one maintains with the relative freedoms of independence.

46. What is the relationship between grief and anxiety?

Grief

a process during which a person mourns the loss of something, whether that be a loved one, a home, or even something less tangible, like self-esteem.

Hurricanes hit; cancer strikes; drunk drivers run over loved ones. Real calamity characterizes life. These losses can devastate, leaving a lifelong impact. We might ask how we will be able to go on, or how to fill such a hole as has been left in the wake of a particular loss. Anxiety is so appropriate because it reflects real, seemingly unspeakable loss. Only the grieving process allows us to slowly restabilize our shattered senses of self.

The kind of loss always shapes the anxiety. Sibling loss can set in motion guilt for the surviving siblings. Not only does one lose a sibling, but one also has to struggle with the actualization of what had been a prior fantasy at times: the natural wish to murder the sibling. These feelings can leave one feeling deserving of punishment and lead to depression, a real punishment. Siblings may then attempt to compensate by becoming hyperresponsible. The death of a parent can also bring people to treatment because it leaves them feeling that they do not know how to go on. Despite their chronological age, they can psychologically return to feelings of childhood vulnerability and of needing a parent so deeply.

As a function of grieving, a person can both let go of the lost parent or sibling as well as incorporate the most treasured aspects of that loved one into one's own personality as a way to move on. The anxiety of death, loss, or separation can be devastating; it can also promote psychological growth in mysterious ways.

47. What if my doctor tells me I will die soon?

Learning that one will die soon can be the most devastating news to hear. Depending on the psychology of the listener, many reactions can follow, ranging from total rage and panic to a type of serenity and pressure to finish one's business in this life. Reading *Tuesdays With Morrie* by Mitch Albom[3] or *Intoxicated By My Illness* by Anatole Broyard[4] can be helpful in making the experience as positive as possible and in negotiating the undeniable loss at hand. Perhaps the strangest experience is feeling well physically and sound mentally but living with the knowledge that a metastatic cancer will soon become lethal.

I believe it becomes paramount to focus on the individual's immediate needs in the context of his or her own psychology. There is no prewritten algorithm to follow in managing death successfully. Each dying person must discover her own. I will tell a patient that I cannot help her with her death, but I can help her with her life; what does she want to do with the time remaining? What business would she like to finish and to whom does she wish to say goodbye? Realizing the finality can precipitate major fears of losing control and not knowing the next step; consultation with a psychiatrist at this moment can be invaluable.

Time takes on new meanings as it becomes finite, perhaps for the first time. As death draws near and physical symptoms emerge, involving a hospice care specialist can address major questions of physical discomfort and the specifics of how a person would like to die, thus reducing the immediate anxieties of pain and end-of-life procedures.

48. How does anxiety appear in a family?

An example might help to introduce some ways in which anxieties within the individuals of a family system can ricochet off of one another to create an inherent anxiety pattern within a given family. The anxiety in one generation can thus transmit to the next.

Imagine one of a family's children dies of a medical illness, thus creating an acute loss for all. The father might remember the grieving or lack of grieving that took place when he lost his sister in childhood; these memories wake up a cascade of anxiety from his own unresolved grief about this loss. They also leave him with longings for the child he has lost. He might try to distance himself from his wife and other children for fear of reexperiencing the loss of his deceased child. He may resort to drinking, thus being like his own father who drank when his sister died. The mother might take blame for the death of the child, blaming her DNA and feeling guilty for the loss of her child from this illness. She, too, may distance herself from the other children so as to protect herself against feelings of loss. She may fight with her husband for distancing himself from her; this distance between the two parents, who are at the top of the family hierarchy, creates a gap between them, as well as the obvious gap between the children and the parents. The children become anxious from this distance, as they are more neglected and get less love and attention than they want.

Survivors of the Holocaust provide many examples of the transmission of one generation's trauma to the next. In these families, where seemingly unspeakable, actual violence, destruction, and calculated eradication took place, many members of the older generation became scarred for life. For many, though they may have survived physiologically, the world may have never felt safe again. It makes sense that this outlook would particularly shape the raising and perceived protection of their own children, perhaps their greatest treasure. On many levels, spoken and not, constant fear, anxiety, and paranoia—conscious and unconscious—characterized attitudes of child rearing. A fear of losing any member of the family often intensified the bond between the existing members. As adults, these offspring often report spending a lifetime recovering from the constant fear which they imagine to be present, fear which their parents instilled in them in the service of protecting them. This fear can make a child's wish to leave, to explore the world on his own terms, to marry someone other than of his ethnic or religious background, or to challenge his parents' authority carry the perception of doing actual harm to the existing family members. These relatives may, in fact, respond to the grown child's actions as being injurious, given the intensity of anxiety provoked at potentially experiencing another loss or perceived loss.

Selma's comments:

Early on, in the beginning of my treatment, I started a long diatribe against myself. I also harped angrily about my husband and about our lack of and poor handling of what scant money we had at a time that he already felt bad enough about our state of affairs. When I was done with my dramatic tirade, I told my analyst that I sounded just like my mother, but that instead of feeling justified by my outburst, I felt devastated by my misery. I imagined he would respond to the core things I had said, if not continue with more criticism.

Instead, he said, "it's good you can see it (referring to my remark about my mother)." At the time, I thought his was a pretty stupid remark, because I had given him a lot of angry material to work with, and now for what? But as usual, I thought about his remark a lot. In a word picture, I had shown him how vile and thoughtless I was to a husband who would give me the world if he were able. Instead of going over that, my analyst chose to honor me with the knowledge that I was able to see something that might be impossible for others to see. This small beginning of self-respect, little by little, over the course of a long time, helped me to see how often I had responded to my own life's situations in my mother's voice. I saw how I held on to my concept of who she was, if not to the worst, martyrlike aspect of her, which did not reflect her whole personality.

My internal responses and self-criticisms were totally inappropriate, as my life was very different in actuality. Sometimes in great despair, I would act like my mother in my self-pity. My analyst might say on a rare occasion, "the hope would be that you could live a better life than your mother was able to," or, "you couldn't live with her, and you couldn't live without her." In time, I could see it myself. First in hindsight, and then remarkably and miraculously to me, I could feel my anxiety and contain it in my throat. I would hold back my remarks, recover in time, and then make an appropriate response to my husband, and especially to my children.

I know my mother was not to blame for it all. Over what seemed like the longest of time, I even came to understand her dilemmas and to have empathy and consideration for her. I became grateful that she had been able to love me as she had. Things took such a shift that in her 90th year, while widowed and losing her friends in another state, I insisted that she move to the city in which I lived. I found a retirement center only blocks away, and my family and I incorporated her daily routines into our lives. I had not seen her so happy in many years, and when she had a stroke, I kept her close to my home and saw her every day for the remaining two years of her life. I came to know the attendants of the home as friends. They commented on our love and on how lonely others those whose families came infrequently to visit were. When my mother passed, I requested that contributions be made in her name to a psychoanalytic foundation. Without this analytic experience of treatment, those years would never have happened in this healthier way. I was then my own person and was able to love her for being my mother. I felt she owed that to my psychoanalysis.

What does all of this have to do with anxiety? The most anxious of times were when I was sure everything would cave in on me. In retrospect, I saw the times when I felt I would not make it were those very times when I was getting better. I gave up using her words and seeing myself as I thought she saw me; I tried to find my own voice. I didn't know how to do it, and my native trust in my own resources was very weak. But it happened. And as it did, my anxiety receded remarkably.

49. How does anxiety appear in children and adolescents?

This book is largely devoted to the anxiety phenomenon experienced in adults. However, children experience at least as much, if not more, anxiety than adults. After all, much adult anxiety has its roots in childhood. Behaviors that would tip parents off to their children's being anxious might include crying, difficulty separating or attending school, difficulty sleeping, wetting the bed, losing control of stool, torturing animals, setting fires, vandalizing property, having an unusual level of sexual curiosity or behavior, exhibiting odd eating behaviors, having an unusual or new preoccupation with weight or body image, or simply telling a parent that they do not feel good about themselves or that they feel nervous in certain situations. Many similar anxieties expose themselves under the framework of adolescence. Anxiety often lies underneath promiscuity, drug experimentation, threatening or violent behavior, poor school performance or shy, inhibited social behavior.

It is worth wondering whether children today are more or less anxious than children of prior generations. When children in this era line up at the summer camp pharmacy to take their antidepressants, something seems to be too anxious about the way they feel. Children can be the worst-treated of any group by their families; it is so easy for the adult mind to disavow the raw, regular daily needs of children who need so much time and guidance. Leaving children without this support creates real feelings of emptiness in children, who then attempt to fill these perceived deficits with abusive relationships, with alcohol, or with overachievement. If, for any reason, you believe your child or adolescent may have anxiety of any type, many resources exist to use as referrals. Two rating scales in the back of this book are for children and adolescents;

references for books and professional psychological testing are to be found in the reference section. Grandparental involvement, tutors at school programs, and the active involvement of others can all do wonders. The first place to start is consultation with a reliable professional.

50. What is the relationship between alcohol and anxiety?

Alcohol is in a category of its own when it comes to anxiety. Not only is alcohol such a common substance of use and abuse in our culture, but it is sufficiently socially acceptable so as to find a presence in Olympics and Super Bowl advertisements. Alcohol serves as a social lubricant in our society; members of our culture use it to prepare for a date, make a professional presentation, make it easier to attend a work function, or before having intercourse. It is usually accurate to say that if alcohol really helps you to feel better, then you probably have anxiety. It is very common for patients to report that alcohol provides a deeply self-soothing state of mind, involving heightened creativity and a heightened sense of integrity. People report that they are feeling at their best when they are drinking—attractive, whole, glamorous, loved, and alive. If, for whatever reason, you find yourself thinking that you drink too much; find yourself annoyed when people ask you about your drinking; have tried to cut back on your own; or find yourself drinking in the morning shortly after you wake up, you may meet criteria for alcohol dependence and would benefit from consultation with a mental health professional. As much as alcohol may make anxiety disappear in the short term, chronic use of and withdrawal from alcohol only makes anxiety worse in the long term.

51. What is the relationship between other drugs and anxiety?

There are so many different drugs of use and abuse in our society; it is impossible to discuss more than a few in this text. Several appear commonly: marijuana, cocaine, heroin, prescription opiates, and ecstasy. These are perhaps the most commonly abused after alcohol in the self-management of anxiety.

Marijuana is a long-standing remedy used not just in this culture, but others historically, to help free people from the anxious chains that bind them. Many report that marijuana helps them to feel more free. It often creates a rebellious feeling, one of feeling able to do whatever one wants (the phenomenon commonly reported in adolescents wanting to belong to a group). Marijuana can allow people to feel that their inner selves are acceptable in a social setting, thus illustrating the basic dynamic of an anxiety disorder—that the feeling of shame that commonly accompanies anxiety is unacceptable.

Cocaine has a similar effect. Often people with post-traumatic stress disorder or the anxiety that stems from depression report that cocaine allows them the energy to stay up all night with friends or lovers talking about many details of their past in a way that feels intimate at the time. Cocaine can create a false sense of energy, security, and intimacy; it often goes along with depression and with the self-medication of depression.

Heroin and other prescription opiates, readily available on the Internet via sham doctors with licenses who make opiates available to anyone for the right price, help people with the anxiety of rage. In my experience, it seems that patients who abuse opiates the most tend to have a primary difficulty with anger, and that the anger, because of its destructive nature, makes them feel unlovable and worthless. However, the opiate also provides a euphoric kind of feeling that recreates feelings of genuine love and belonging. A colleague of mine who works with heroin addicts reports that up to 85% of the opiate addicts whom she treats have been sexually abused. It is not surprising that these patients would create or seek a medium through which they could gratify their appetite for love, but yet do so via a drug that involves no human contact.

Perhaps the most popular anxiety drug of abuse would be ecstasy, also known as the "love drug." Patients who have used ecstasy at parties and overnight raves often describe feelings of absolute euphoria, love, belonging, and connectedness. They feel safe touching and loving each other, staring at each other's genitalia, or sensing a blissful, babylike kind of safety in the world. That ecstasy works so well to dissolve anxiety in the short term is entirely compatible with what we know of serotonin's impact in the treatment of anxiety. Ecstasy increases serotonin quickly and provides immediate relief. The serotonin medicines do so over weeks, with a similar, but a more muted, effect. It is important to keep in mind that ecstasy, like the reported positive effects of many drugs, provides only an artifice of intimacy. In fact, while people feel they are loving and sharing, they might also be acquiring sexually transmitted diseases or going home with partners they later regret having gone home with. Other users report grinding their teeth, developing high fevers, "disco dumping" (defecating in their pants), or ending up in a hospital from its effects on the body, none of which seems so desirable or loving.

52. What is the relationship between anxiety and depression?

Often, patients come to my office complaining of anxiety, and the more I listen to them, the more I realize they are in the middle of a full-blown depression, with anxiety and sadness as the major symptoms. The fear of bad things happening dominates the mental landscape. Someone may fear going crazy. She may fear being left. She may fear bad things happening to her or to her family. She may fear being unable to provide for her family in the future. She may fear an inability to function and to sustain a life for herself. Or she may fear experiencing an unbearable psychic pain.

It is important to explain depression, briefly. Commonly spanning at least a two-week period, depression includes feeling low sex drive, decreased interest in life, increased **rumination** or sense of guilt, low energy, low mood, deep feelings of the blues, sadness, inability to rally, poor concentration ability, low appetite, decreased food intake, feelings of paralysis or heaviness, contemplation of suicide, and/or a basic listless quality. Life may simply no longer feel worthwhile or worth living. It is not surprising that one of the most common elements of depression is anxiety. There are many ways to think about this relationship, and much thought has been given to this clinically. Often, a loss or a sad event takes place, either real or perceived. This injury, in turn, triggers the depressive feelings. Not attaining one's desired status can leave one feeling less

Rumination

the process of going over and over the same thought in one's mind to the exclusion of other thoughts and without any clear benefit.

than ideal; this loss of ideal opens the floodgates of depression.

Anxiety stemming from depression can mushroom into the panic of hopelessness, which, in turn, can lead to frenetic behavioral attempts to manage the anxiety with impulsive decisions. At the time, these desperate attempts seem to provide relief, but longitudinally, they can trigger further distress. For example, a patient who is acutely anxious about future terrorist attacks may decide to pack the family apartment, leave her spouse, and move the family to a rural setting. Once she relocated and thought the distress was confined to the urban landscape, this patient's untreated depression might manifest further anxious symptoms. Now she may believe that the water supply of the town will be contaminated or preoccupy herself with rural terrorist attacks. This impulsive streak might make a doctor suspect bipolar illness (manic depression); however, often action-prone plans stem from the anxiety fueled by an untreated depression. Anxiety is a major piece of the larger clinical picture so common today. Now, in as much panic as before, the patient is isolated and without the social and community resources familiar from years in her former neighborhood. You can see how the cycle worsens without treatment.

I have thought of this particular anxiety as reflecting a question within the self. Will the individual be able to return to an ideal sense of self? Anxiety serves as the substrate of this preoccupation. The internal anxiety, after a patient has been fired, might be, "will I be able to work and maintain a job at the level I did before?" This initial worry can spring into anxiety over survival. This metamorphosis creates a vulnerable state, which, if not mended, can reinforce further depression. It is not surprising that as one's depression gets treated, anxiety invariably lessens.

Rick's comments:

It's not always easy to tell, even about oneself, where one symptom ends and another symptom begins. At least I don't find it easy and I doubt that I'm alone in this. I tend to think of my depressive tendencies as involving lethargy, sadness, a lack of enjoyment in life and a sense of being very alone and disinterested. Anxiety, for me, is more of a jittery feeling—more alive than the depressive ones, more active— yet not in a comfortable way. Maybe it makes sense to say that my depression is more like pain, my anxiety more like an itch, and my OCD like an attempt to scratch that itch.

53. What is the anxiety of suicide?

Suicide is a highly complicated psychiatric phenomenon; I often see it as falling into five major categories. The first would be an impulsive act in a person with a highly self-destructive nature who becomes disinhibited enough through the use of alcohol—or another method leading to a lack of impulse control—which allows him to act on the actual pain he feels in life. In this situation, the anxiety is that of intense psychic pain and a wish to rid oneself of it. Victims of incest, survivors of overwhelming trauma, or end-of-life patients might be examples of those who struggle with fantasies of hopelessness or worthlessness that take the risk of acting on them one day.

The second is that person who realizes at some level that he is becoming psychotic or having a break with reality—he knows he is beginning to lose his mind.

Patients describe this mind-shattering experience as profoundly disturbing, especially to someone who realizes some version of what he is losing. It is not uncommon for such patients to try to kill themselves. The anxiety may be a sense of annihilation or fragmentation which feels beyond repair. To leave this panic, a patient in this state might impulsively jump off the roof, out the window, or off of a bridge.

The third is the chronically suicidal patient. This patient spends years thinking of suicide and keeping suicidal thoughts and feelings a secret. It seems that this kind of patient feels trapped in a life of pain. Therefore, thinking of suicide serves as a way out, an option or escape hatch from the pain and seemingly enslaved nature of life. One day, often for reasons we will never know, the person decides to make fantasy a reality.

A fourth major category is the patient who has become majorly depressed. Symptoms can be an absolute wish not to wake up, a profound sense of hopelessness, or an inability to visualize life's going on. These patients can develop an impulsive pressure to kill themselves. The anxiety in these situations is similar to that of **psychosis**, in that the patient is suffering from a kind of pain that seems insurmountable. However, this anxiety represents distorted thinking. Patients who accidentally survived jumping from the Golden Gate Bridge all reported that they knew they had made a mistake the second they jumped.

Psychosis
a state of thinking in which reality is distorted in a severe way.

The last category is the patient who receives bad news, possibly news of a worsening or progressive medical condition. These patients, it seems, become suicidal as a way to try to manage the overwhelming pain and anxiety that they are feeling in the moment.

One feature that we see clinically is that oftentimes the patient who is able to speak about wanting to kill herself is at least ambivalent about it. She leaves genuine room for intervention, but the person who feels deeply ashamed of his wish and is unable to speak with anyone about it might jump or shoot himself before anyone has had a chance to intervene.

Anxiety is central to all of these types of suicide. Taking anxiety seriously and obtaining the right treatment can prevent suicide. If you are in an urgent situation, call 911 or 1-800-SUICIDE. Help is always available, and options other than killing yourself always exist.

54. What is the anxiety of psychosis?

Psychosis, generally speaking, is a type of loss of reality testing; properly speaking, it is a disorder of or a problem with thinking. This shift in thinking can be one of the most difficult anxieties for a patient to confront because of the overwhelming sense of loss. The psychotic process can be transient or long-term. Transient causes of psychosis include substance abuse, an acute delirium from a medication, or a medical condition such as an infection or a new onset tumor. It can also be in the context of a worsening mood disorder, such as depression or bipolar illness. At times, anxiety can, in and of itself, become psychotic as seen in extreme obsessive-compulsive disorders or eating disorders. Finally, there is the psychosis of more primary disorders of thought such as schizophrenia or schizoaffective disorder. The experience is commonly described as feeling a shattering loss of control, an overwhelming sense of despair, or an extreme futility. Much of this anxiety can be soothed, either by receiving medication or seeking the structural intervention of hospitalization.

55. What if I can't stop thinking about the way I look?

Body **dysmorphia** is a feeling that something with one's body is not right. This process focuses on a feeling of one's nose being too large or too short, one being too fat or too skinny, one's legs not feeling the right length or right width, or, perhaps, feeling that one's penis is not large enough or that one's breasts are too small. These self-perceptions can, when contrasted with the overvalued ideals of our culture, drive much of America's **obsession** with cosmetic surgery. The problem, of course, is that the real issue is not the body itself, but the mind's perception of the body. This symptom—viewing something about one's body as defective—serves as a reservoir to house other feelings of defectiveness that one has about oneself or one's sense of security in the world. For example, the woman who sees fat and her own perceived fat as disgusting often feels, consciously or unconsciously, that she is disgusting.

Patients with body dysmorphia harbor the illusion that if they can only fix their perceived defect, then they will feel fixed in their personality. But once the nose is repaired in a surgical intervention, patients with body dysmorphia often discover a new defective feature of their body on which to focus. This pattern of obsession keeps the experience of criticism alive; it reinforces the patient's negative self-worth. In a most common scenario, a woman looking at herself in a mirror simply

Dysmorphia
the idea that one's body (or parts of one's body) looks much worse or deformed than it actually is.

Obsession
a repetitive, intrusive thought that is difficult for one to get rid of, despite a knowledge that the thought is unreasonable.

87

cannot tell if she is skinny or fat. Her need to use a scale to measure her weight parallels her kind of emotional numbness. As she cannot tell whether she is skinny or fat, she also cannot tell whether she is happy, sad, anxious, blue, or excited. This obsession provides an externalized avenue through which to contain, to think about, and to connect with feelings of badness and defectiveness about oneself. Hence, the abusive cycle repeats itself.

56. Does anxiety connect the mind and the body?

Commonly known as somatization, the body and brain work together in an integral way to illustrate a complicated interface between the mind and the body. Anxiety often is at the root of this interface. We know that, neurobiologically, the anxiety system is linked to the rest of the brain through other central parts called the hypothalamus and the pituitary gland. These regions, when anxious, fire multiple kinds of hormones, including cortisol, epinephrine, and norepinephrine within the body. These hormones travel down the vagus nerve and hit all of the major organ systems, including the head (headache); the voice (the raised-pitch voice); the jaw (**TMJ**, teeth grinding); the lungs (shortness of breath); the heart (palpitations); the gut (diarrhea, constipation, and nausea and/or vomiting); the back (pain); the limbs (trembling); or the peripheral nervous system (sweating and shaking). When some people are feeling anxious, their brains convert this emotional sensation into the physical experiences of nausea, aches, pains, numbness, contractions of the uterus, or hives of the skin. This transaction serves as one of the body's ways to display its anxiety. It is very difficult for

TMJ

Temporomandibular joint. The joint that connects the jaw to the skull.

patients to believe that the original problem itself might be anxiety, since they actually experience physical distress.

After ruling out the major causes of any kind of medical problem and an appropriate referral to a psychiatrist, careful history can reveal links between the mind and the body and allow one to address the mental component involved in the physical display of these symptoms. Physical discomfort can represent an unusual way of remembering a past bodily or emotional experience. For example, a man who had asthma as a young boy could find himself with an asthmatic attack on the anniversary of the death of his mother— a way to remember and memorialize her death through shortness of breath, which might be a more emotionally acceptable version of crying. In classic examples of conversion disorder, a patient might experience paralysis of his right arm at a time he wants to punch his boss; or an entire group of Laotian women who witnessed the massacre of their families might develop blindness for the rest of their lives, despite normal functioning of the nerves and retinas of their visual systems.

57. How does anxiety show itself in generalized pain, back pain, or irritable bowel syndrome?

Pain is a highly subjective symptom, which has both psychological and physiologic causes. Back pain serves as the classic example of the multidetermined nature of pain. However, numerous examples exist. Anyone who has worked with pain or experienced pain knows that it is not correlated just to the level of tissue

MRI

Magnetic resonance imaging. A type of imaging in which parts of the body, such as the brain, are visualized in much more detail than on a CAT scan.

pathology. For example, consider 100 patients with objective findings on **MRIs** of their spines. It is not possible to correlate the level of tissue pathology observable on MRI with the level of pain that a patient experiences. Similarly, people can experience nausea as a way to contain their anxiety. This nausea infrequently leads to vomiting, but the fear of losing control and the pain and concern that come from the nausea are just as prominent. Psychotherapy in these cases addresses whatever component of the pain might be anxiety-laden. Patients with back pain, for example, often report that as they are able to identify their anger, their back pain itself lessens. Or, patients who have suffered bad menstrual cramps report after 6 months of psychotherapy that their disturbance of menstrual functioning may still be present, but that it does not bother them nearly as much as it did before.

IBS

Irritable bowel syndrome. A group of symptoms, often associated with anxiety and more frequently found in women, that involves abdominal pain, constipation, diarrhea, and other gastrointestinal complaints without any clear medical reason.

Irritable bowel syndrome (IBS) is an extremely common condition in which the patient experiences—without any other acute gastrointestinal pathology—a variety of intestinal or abdominal symptoms, including but not limited to pain, bloating, cramping, and constipation and/or diarrhea. Interestingly enough, the patients who have been diagnosed with irritable bowel syndrome do have, at an actual tissue level, abnormal neuronal functioning which can create the overactivity or underactivity of their gut. However, any clinician who has worked with patients suffering from irritable bowel syndrome or any patient who lives with irritable bowel syndrome knows that there is a clear connection between anxiety and the gut.

The gastrointestinal nervous system (the gut) contains one third the number of nerve cells as does the entire central nervous system (brain and spinal cord), which

90

includes the brain and spinal cord. The brain chemical serotonin, which is central to the body's regulation of anxiety, plays a major role in gastrointestinal function as well. So, there are many good reasons physiologically that anxiety and the chemicals that mediate anxiety also have a major impact on gastrointestinal functioning. Any patient with IBS will tell you that he notices particular specific reactions between his anxiety and his bowel functioning. Some patients will report that during times of stress they become acutely constipated; others will report not being able to control their diarrhea. Many things can be done through seeing the gastroenterologist, including adding certain kinds of medications or making changes in diet. However, it is always important for a patient with irritable bowel syndrome to consult at least with a psychiatrist to discuss treatment options from a psychiatric and psychotherapeutic point of view. Medications in the Serotonin Reuptake Inhibitor (SRI) family can alter the constipation as well as treat the anxiety, while some of the older tricyclic antidepressants can manage both the diarrhea and the anxiety.

58. Can anxiety ever make me feel that I am not real?

Commonly known as dissociation, overwhelming anxiety can precipitate symptoms of loss of time or sense of personality. Usually, patients realize it has happened after the fact. For example, a patient may miss three subway stops before realizing that she needed to get off three stops back. Another example would be a man who hears his friends talk about a night where they all celebrated, but he has no conscious memory of the event. A woman who experiences herself talking to you from the perspective of herself looking down at the two of you having the conversation is yet another example. Dissociation is one of the body's responses to overwhelming anxiety—it takes the conscious mind out of the actuality of the moment. Perhaps this strategy reflects a survival tool that helped a child who was suffering from neglect or abuse create a belief that the abuse was happening to someone else while he watched, thus creating a sense that the abuse was not actually occurring to him. These moments of dissociation can occur both outside of therapy or within the session itself; either way, the precipitating trigger is one of anxiety. Learning to identify the anxiety as it emerges can, over time, help to prevent the need for the dissociation. More importantly, it can provide access to the walled off, unconsciously buried painful emotional memories that are so intimately connected to the patient's conscious experiences of anxiety or panic.

The most profound examples of dissociation are either the fugue state or the multiple personality disorder. Occasionally you might read in the newspaper a story similar to that of a man who "woke up" in the hospital three weeks from his last conscious memory, only to learn that over that time period he had invented a new identity for himself and gone back to the state where he did his military training. While there, he attempted to reengage in training maneuvers on base, only to be discovered in the woods wearing fatigues and face paint. The history might then reveal that his marriage was crumbling and that he had recently been fired from his job. In the extreme form, patients can shift between alternating personalities ("alters") without awareness of the distinction between the two. These patient histories invariably have detailed accounts of overwhelming abuse, which then leads to such overwhelming anxiety that the brain splits the mind of the person off from that anxiety via the invention of a new personality.

59. How is lying connected to anxiety?

Lying—the conscious attempt to manipulate the truth in order to deceive the listener—often stems from anxiety. We try to hide that of which we are ashamed, and that of which we are ashamed generates anxiety. Hence we lie about affairs we have had or cheating we have done so as to avoid the shame of owning those feelings and having our actions made known to others in our community. Perhaps even the mind's defense mechanisms—like denial or rationalization—are ways to lie to ourselves to protect ourselves from a greater truth. A painkiller addict may lie to himself by saying that he takes pills in order to feel love and bliss but hide from himself the truth: that he wants to destroy himself because he feels so worthless, just as he felt his parents hated him for his lack of perfect behavior when he was a kid. It is not surprising that most lie detector tests in history, like the polygraph, draw their scientific evidence from the measurement of physiologic signs of anxiety, such as pulse rate, respiration rate, sweating rate, and blood pressure.

60. What is generalized anxiety disorder?

Generalized anxiety disorder usually comes across in the patient who does not worry about any one topic or fear in particular, but instead always characteristically worries. It is a free-floating anxiety that might be described as a mosquito that cannot be swatted, or a background noise that cannot be turned off. The anxiety switches back and forth from one topic to the next.

A generalized anxiety sufferer might worry about the latest airplane crash, switch to the next terrorist attack, return to his boss's reaction to his latest business report, focus on the redness on his arm as indicative of a likely first sign of cancer, fret over the weather turning bad for tomorrow's party, and then focus on a feeling that he has now become too heavy from eating that donut. Generalized anxiety disorder in its purest form seems to suggest a basic level of not feeling safe in the world. It also reinforces someone's feeling very important. If he has to think about everything so much that his thoughts are central to every action, then he must indeed be very powerful and in control of the universe. He must compromise when including someone else or some level of risk in a situation while also keeping very alive the possibility that the other person's involvement could lead to a bad outcome.

61. What is hypochondriasis?

Hypochondriasis

an exaggerated fear that one has an illness or disease based on a misinterpretation of a bodily symptom and without any medical basis.

Hypochondriasis is an anxiety that manifests itself in and around the body. The patient with hypochondriasis constantly fears and believes that any bodily symptom that he or she experiences is attributable to a serious and/or malignant medical illness. A patient with hypochondriasis fears that she will die from this medical condition or she has a medical condition that is not diagnosable with appropriate clinical or physical examination and/or laboratory findings. This anxiety can take over the life of the patient's mind. A hypochondriac with a pimple on his penis believes it can become a lethal, sexually transmitted disease. A numbness on the finger can cause concern that it is the first symptom of a brain tumor. Nausea can be interpreted as stemming from ovarian cancer, and that worry, like in any other condition, can mushroom into an all-consuming pattern. The evaluation and management of hypochondriasis usually responds best to regular visits with an internist or family medicine doctor who can reassure the patient, over time, that he is not dying. However, psychological treatment—if these anxious patients are willing to engage in it—can be markedly helpful. The key is to try to help the person see that the discomfort that she is feeling stems from anxiety rather than from a bodily condition, and to then focus on the patient's need to create the anxiety rather than the actual somatic disturbance. Oftentimes, there will be a history in the family of someone who has been sick and has received love and attention for being sick. The patient then has a learned behavior of obtaining gratification by being in the sick role. It may create "legitimate" attention for a patient who does not attend a given family function, or it may be a means to get attention that otherwise would not be permissible in a family system. For example, a patient who harbors longstanding resentment and jealousy towards a sibling but knows that displays of frustration and aggression will only create family havoc might unwittingly find themselves in an emergency room on the day of the sibling's graduation from college, being evaluated again for a brain tumor after experiencing a migraine headache.

62. What is obsessive-compulsive disorder?

Obsessive-compulsive disorder is characterized by intensive obsessions and/or **compulsions** which patients experience and which absolutely interfere with workings of their minds and lives. Obsessions are commonly known as worries, fears, thoughts, or feelings that one cannot stop thinking about. Hearing

Compulsion
a behavior, such as washing one's hands multiple times an hour, in response to an obsessive thought.

95

musical passages, counting numbers, or repeating words over and over again may be other avenues of the anxiety's expression. A compulsion, on the other hand, is a ritual that one performs to undo the fear that one experiences from the obsession. For example, if someone becomes intensely fearful of being dirty, then she might have the compulsion of washing her hands. If someone becomes fearful that he will set the apartment on fire, so he will combat the fear by repeatedly returning to the apartment to check the stove, etc., only to then do it all over again. Obsessive-compulsive disorder is not to be confused with an obsessive personality style found in someone who likes things to be arranged in a particular way or to be in control of any given project. Obsessive-compulsive disorder is a much higher level of private obsession and/or compulsion, which impairs someone's life. In addition to impairing function, it can disintegrate a family structure inasmuch as family members become hostage to the patient's symptoms. For example, if a patient insists that food be washed in a particular way, hours and hours can be spent with the preparation of a meal. Obsessive-compulsive disorder is generally treatable or at least manageable with the right kind of medication. However, understanding the context in which symptoms arise can also provide huge therapeutic relief. Patients often report experiencing the heightening of their obsessive-compulsive symptoms just as they feel an overwhelming flood of rage. So, it makes sense to consider the obsession as a method to distract the person from the very rage that he so feels and fears. Likewise, a connection between sexual urges and obsessive-compulsive preoccupation with the perceived dangerous consequences of acting on these sexual urges occurs time and again. Understanding these links can deepen both psychotherapeutic engagement and benefit.

Rick's comments:

My OCD rituals mostly revolve around attempts to keep myself safe despite actions that I take that are self-destructive and dangerous. If I eat a very sugary dessert even though I am a diabetic, I might repeat the phrase "I'll try to do better" every time I stand up or sit down. Do I really believe that this will keep me safe? No. Then again, a baseball pitcher who makes certain that he doesn't step on the white lines as he runs off the field doesn't really believe that this will make his curve ball better; he does it as an attempt to gain additional control over his situation, to gain an edge beyond what his talent provides. Since it is easy for the player to avoid touching the lines, there is no risk of failing to fulfill this ritual and thus losing his "advantage" over the hitter. This is not OCD—it's a simple, doable ritual which does not intrude on the player's ability to function. What, however, if the white-lines skipping was only the beginning? What if the pitcher, in order to feel in control or safe, has to always throw curveballs to left-handed hitters, fastballs down the middle of the plate to right-handed hitters and only high pitches from the fifth inning on while the thought "I must not give up a home run" swirls endlessly around in his mind and he must avoid looking at the shortstop and left fielder during even innings. This is how OCD can intrude on, even ravage, a life, and it's what people coping with OCD, including me, go through on a day-to-day basis. That's why it's good to know—very good to know—that it is treatable.

63. What is social phobia?

Social phobia is, in its essence, an extreme fear of social interactions. It can be experienced as being scared of riding the elevator at work, going on a date,

The Many Faces of Anxiety

eating in public, or presenting at a work conference. The patient expects the worst possible outcome. The life history of such a patient might involve a highly critical or substance-abusing parent who became disinhibited and then attacked the patient when she was a young child. Perhaps these attacks occurred while the child did exciting things. The patient learned to associate feeling anxious with feeling excited. Social phobia, therefore, creates a kind of a compromise. The patient can keep a critical parent alive in her mind by keeping herself inhibited from progressing in life. While she recreates and remembers these painful times, she also keeps the hopes alive of rising in life (the elevator), sharing intimacy with close friends over a meal (the date or eating in public), or exhibiting her natural talents (the conference presentation), hopes about which all children regularly talk and fantasize.

64. What is a specific phobia?

Generally speaking, phobia means fear. A specific phobia can be anything from a fear of the number 13 to a fear of needles to a fear of snakes to a fear of heights. Many of the same principles that apply to one phobia apply to another. A couple of the most common phobias serve as examples to illustrate these ideas. For example, the passenger with a flying phobia experiences absolute horror at the idea of being trapped on an airplane. This fear can handicap one's ability to take business trips by airplane or can cause one to prohibit family members from flying. A flying phobia may have many roots, but often it involves a basic difficulty trusting the world or trusting others with one's safety.

In a more psychological approach, simply exploring what comes to the patient's mind around flying and inquiring about sexual desires and/or fears that the patient potentially struggled with at the time of the flying phobia's onset can provide symptom relief. If a woman can connect her conscious fear of the plane's crashing with an unconscious fear of being punished for wishing to be sexual on the trip on which the phobia commenced, then the conscious symptom can disappear. Others might experience a genuine fear of success, or of climbing to new heights in their lives. A man might have panic attacks on the plane in conjunction with the feeling of permanently leaving home, marrying, or taking an exciting trip. This sensed loss of control can have sexual associations, in that the man can feel that the excitement of going higher is linked (often unconsciously) with sexual aspirations. If this man can connect his conscious fear of blowing up while on the plane with his feelings of his sexual or financial potency (and his fears of sexual or financial success), then flying on business trips might immediately feel less threatening. Other strategies, such as medication or behavioral treatments, can provide immediate symptom management (see Part III, Treatment).

In claustrophobia (literally, fear of the claustrum, or mother's womb), one becomes overwhelmingly fearful of being trapped in a closed space and being unable to get out. This fear can link to fantasies of being trapped on a bridge or in a tunnel. However, fears of going on a date, being stuck in a movie theater, riding in a car without being the driver, or receiving treatment in a hospital or clinic setting often elicit panic attacks or anxious reactions. These psychological claustrophobias might recreate an experience from earlier in life when the patient felt overwhelmed and sensed that she could not get out of a trapped situation or away from a certain person, such as from her mother or family, or from an abusive relationship. Again, in almost any case, these extremely common phobias are treatable (see Part III, Treatment).

PANIC DISORDER, AGORAPHOBIA
65. What is a panic attack?

A panic attack occurs usually as a seemingly out-of-the-blue sensation that transforms into an overwhelming, crippling, emotional tidal wave of nervousness. Panic attacks have both mental and physical symptoms. Mental symptoms include a fear of doom, worry that something horrible will happen, an overwhelming sense of dread, or an immediate sense of pending death.

Physical symptoms include chest pain, chest tightness, numbness, tingling, nausea, sweating, or a feeling of nearly passing out. The panic attack, if experienced regularly in the same situation or with a consistent frequency, can progress to what is known as panic disorder. The circumstances surrounding the panic attack can take on a life of their own, thereby becoming hallmark triggers for further attacks. So, if someone has a panic attack driving on the highway in the car, he may come to fear driving on the highway in association with the panic attack. He may then believe that the highway itself or the situation of driving caused the panic attack, rather than whatever underlying anxiety he experienced or was experiencing at the time. A panic attack serves as the body's responding to the mind's inability to handle an overwhelming feeling. With close psychotherapeutic investigation, we usually discover that the panic attack only appeared to occur out of the blue, while a clear, identified stressor, which, up until that point, had been largely unknown to the patient emerges. Close exploration of the circumstances and the feelings surrounding a panic attack help identify the root of the patient's suffering. In its worst-case scenario, panic disorder will lead to agoraphobia, or a "fear of open spaces." This designation means that the patient might become reclusive or stay at home to avoid any situation in which she fears the unforgettable misery of panic attack may recur.

ACUTE STRESS DISORDER AND POSTTRAUMATIC STRESS DISORDER

66. *What is the role of trauma in the creation of anxiety?*

This question raises complicated, far-reaching, and deeply compelling issues. Asking one question in this area raises even more questions than it provides definite answers. However, both **acute trauma** (e.g. being in a car wreck or another near-death situation) and longer-term, lower-grade **strain trauma** (e.g. living over time in an abusive household) can serve as points of departure in beginning to answer this question. Both acute and strain traumas can lead to acute stress disorder or the creation of an anxious personality style.

Acute trauma
immediate, intense, possibly life-threatening situations that can create overwhelming anxiety (e.g. being in a car wreck; performing active duty combat; being raped).

Strain trauma
longer-term, less immediately life-threatening situations that, over time, can create overwhelming anxiety (e.g. living in a violent household).

101

Acute stress disorder and posttraumatic stress disorder can look the same, although they differ in their time frames. Technically, any acute trauma that leads to the symptoms of hyperarousal (including palpitations, racing heart beat, and sweating), reexperiencing (where one experiences **flashbacks**), or avoidance of anything associated with the trauma within thirty days is called acute stress disorder. Those whose symptoms persist beyond thirty days qualify for diagnosis of posttraumatic stress disorder. These distinctions are both interesting and meaningful from a clinical perspective. However, anyone in the midst of these symptoms knows that sensitivity to one's perspective, attempted understanding of one's distress, and the provision of a safe haven to rest are more important than any diagnostic time frame parameters. Exploring emotional reactions related to the trauma in any longer-term healing way happens over time as the sufferer feels safe enough to begin this process. If you wish to learn more about these topics, start with Dr. Judith Herman's *Trauma and Recovery*[5] or Dr. Leonard Shengold's *Soul Murder*.[6]

In cases of torture, we find overwhelming, ghastly, seemingly unspeakable consequences. James Bond may (unrealistically) be tortured on film and recover to a high level of functioning, almost making the notion of torture glamorous via Bond's superherolike defiance of human fear. Examples of torture are unfortunately all too common among military personnel, prisoners of war, or seekers of political asylum from dictatorial societies. Several major components characterize this torture. First, the physical creation of pain is inter-

Flashbacks

a phenomena, usually seen in posttraumatic stress disorder (PTSD), in which a person has the sensation of reexperiencing a particular trauma.

spersed by design with caretaking, as well as with an overt, calculated plan to control the victim's thoughts, to dominate one's thinking, or to brainwash the mind's total functioning. These tactics systematically disintegrate human mental functioning and sense of personal self, a process that has been called "soul murder."

Child abuse, rape, or other sexual crimes might, likewise, result in acute or posttraumatic stress. The example of sexual abuse and the histories of its victims serves as one, among many, example that illustrates general principles of anxiety that stems from trauma. Victims of sexual abuse, whether disorders from incest or from another perpetrator, often feel particularly unprotected and vulnerable. Their overwhelming secret and the sense of shame they carry in keeping the abuse secret make symptoms even more uncomfortable.

Understanding the roots of this shame proves as individual a pursuit as the sufferer is an individual, with his or her own complex life history. Keeping an abuse history secret helps to avoid the perceived fear or humiliation one expects if he or she were to reveal his or her sexual involvement with a forbidden mentor, teacher, relative, or parent. Sharing such histories of abuse might mean reexperiencing feelings of vulnerability or memories of being taken advantage of; or it might mean exposing what feels like an illegal yearning or hunger for affection. Often, victims struggle when revealing that they enjoyed part of the sexual attention they received by their perpetrators, perhaps knowing that such attention felt better than being alone. It takes immense courage to speak aloud of the secrets of sexual abuse. Often, men and women wait decades—suffering privately—before coming forward with their secrets. This courage then allows for repair and safety to take root, both of which can encourage the shame and its attached discomfort to diminish.

In sexual abuse, as in all kinds of torture, an absolute violation of a human boundary occurs such that the world may no longer feel like a safe place. Instead, an actual blurring of the boundary between fantasy and reality emerges. Whereas a normal child may fantasize being sexually involved with his significant caretakers or other adults around him, normative development allows a child to differentiate between fantasy and reality. However, sexual abuse may leave a child not knowing where reality ends or where fantasy starts. This history can make the very nature of fantasy traumatic and invite the possibility that even sexual fantasies could become dangerous inasmuch as they might feel like crossing a forbidden boundary.

Sexual abuse can trigger many different types of anxiety. Patients with phobias, such as needle or tunnel phobias, panic disorder, or eating disorders may have experienced sexual abuse, as may have 50% of those diagnosed with borderline personality disorder. Patients with pain disorders and medical syndromes such as vaginismus (a contracting of the vaginal muscles making penetration of the penis impossible) may have been victims of sexual abuse. Drug abuse, suicide, sexual inhibitions, promiscuity, and sadistic and masochistic personalities also come to mind in contemplating the myriad effects sexual abuse can have in the shaping of a personality.

The anxiety of regular sexual abuse or of regular screaming, yelling, fighting, or witnessing of physical abuse at home can create chronic feelings of insecurity. A man may fear that he will never grow out of being a boy, or a woman may feel trapped as a girl in her adult life. It is not uncommon for patients in the context of trauma to feel both a physical sense of numbness and an emotional lack of reactivity. Numbness, or not feeling things in the body as someone otherwise might, could manifest itself as a loss of genital sensation or as decreased sensation in one's hands. Alternatively, someone may notice that he has a decreased ability to identify his mood, which might actually serve a protective function. Anyone who has read Albert Camus's book *The Stranger*[7] or who has seen the emotional blunting of the abused character in the movie *Mystic River*[8] can appreciate the haunting and deadening of mood that characterize survivors of sexual abuse and posttraumatic stress disorder.

67. What is Xenophobia?

In this current climate of war, the fear of strangers has reached a new peak. A major U.S. national concern has unfolded since September 11, 2001, involving anyone belonging to a Middle Eastern culture. In this case, a real trauma did occur, and our nation, rightfully, is anxious about another attack. However, this anxiety can magnify into xenophobia, a fear of anyone foreign—Middle Easterners, in this case. It can also make people question whom we can trust when we cannot see the enemy. The nation's response has paralleled that of someone who experiences an individual trauma; expecting the worst outcome in any situation

105

inasmuch as a stimulus associated with trauma might lead to the fear of another attack. Fear of strangers provides an excellent way of letting the mind split the world into good and bad, safe and dangerous. It also allows us to forget or deny that we, too, might be doing something bad. Many individuals who have endured a trauma exercise hypervigilance, mentally reexperience the trauma, or sense chronic numbness. In reaction to the terrorist attacks, the nation has done that through its code orange alerts, its repeated images of planes crashing into the World Trade Center, and a wish to avoid the memories of what has happened.

Notes

1. Goleman, D. (2000). Emotional Intelligence. In Sadock, B.J. & Sadock, V.A. (Eds.), *Kaplan and Sadock's comprehensive textbook of psychiatry, Vol. 1.* Philadelphia: Lippincott Williams & Wilkins.

2. Bronson, P. (2002). *What should I do with my life? The true story of people who answered the ultimate question.* New York: Random House.

3. Albom, M. (1997). *Tuesdays with Morrie: An old man, a young man, and life's greatest lesson.* New York: Doubleday.

4. Broyard, A. (1992). *Intoxicated by my illness: And other writings on life and death.* New York: C. Potter.

5. Herman, J. (1997). *Trauma and recovery.* New York: Basic Books.

6. Shengold, L. (1989). *Soul murder: The effects of childhood abuse and deprivation.* New Haven: Yale University Press.

7. Camus, A. (1982). *The stranger.* Trans. Griffith, K. Washington, DC: University Press of America.

8. *Mystic river.* (2003). Clint Eastwood, Director. Based on the novel by Dennis Lehane.

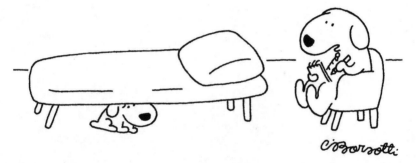

"And what do you think will happen if you <u>do</u> get on the couch?"

Reprinted with permission from The Cartoon Bank, a division of *The New Yorker* magazine.

PART THREE

Treatment

What is the difference between a psychiatrist and a psychologist, between a social worker and a nurse? Whom should I see?

What are the most important things to find out from my doctor when I am figuring out a treatment course?

What are the different kinds of therapies?

More...

68. What is the difference between a psychiatrist and a psychologist, between a social worker and a nurse? Whom should I see?

Mental health professionals have varying degrees of training, but with so many avenues open to become a therapist and with so many people claiming to be therapists, it makes sense to understand these differences and to get the treatment that is right for you. A psychiatrist is a physician, meaning that he or she is a **medical doctor (MD)**, went to medical school, and can both prescribe medication and understand the interaction of your medicine with other health problems and/or medications you may be taking. A psychiatrist might also practice psychotherapy, though many insurance plans today only cover a psychiatrist if the patient needs to be on medication. Feel free to ask your psychiatrist what kinds of therapy he or she practices. If you do need to be on a medication, working with a psychiatrist who also does skilled psychotherapy makes life a lot simpler because you can receive the medication and the therapy under one roof. A psychiatrist can also be a **doctor of osteopathy (D.O.)**, which includes slightly different medical training.

A psychologist has graduate training in clinical psychology (if she sees patients)—either a master's degree or PhD degree. Psychologists have extensive training in brain science, models of the mind, psychiatric diagnosis, psychologic diagnosis, learning theory and disorders, psychological and/or neuropsychiatric testing, and often excellent clinical training. Their practice is usually limited to diagnosis, therapy, and psychological testing; feel free to ask what kinds of therapy they practice.

MD

Medical doctor. The degree that all physicians attain after successfully completing four years of medical school.

D.O.

Doctor of Osteopathy. The degree that physicians who study osteopathy, or a system of medicine that studies the effects of the musculo-skeletal system on the rest of the body, obtain after four years of medical school.

A social worker practices therapy with a master's degree or a PhD in social work. His or her clinical training provides a relatively faster entry to clinical practice, but many have done further subspecialization in certain types of therapy and can administer these therapies as well as anyone. With so many types of training, it becomes less about one's degree as about the intelligence and experience of the practitioner.

A psychiatric nurse can fall into different categories: **registered nurse (RN), licensed practical nurse (LPN),** or nurse practitioner (MNS).

The exact training of your therapist is important, and you should feel free to ask about his or her credentials. Perhaps more important than the credentials *per se* is his or her experience in treating your type of anxiety. One of the most important factors is your feeling in the room with this person. Your comfort as the patient and your sense of this person's ability to help you are critical factors in choosing a therapist. If there is some question as to whether you feel taken seriously or as to the appropriateness of fit with your therapist, do not hesitate to ask for a second opinion. If there is any question about your diagnosis, find a reputable psychiatrist who can figure out the subtle intricacies of your condition and make a proper diagnosis. Remember that your mind is a part of your body, and therapists get in trouble diagnosing anxiety but forgetting that a medical condition might complicate or explain a patient's mental distress. A psychiatrist can also discuss the use of medication with you to assess the risks versus benefits of a trial period. Practitioners who have trained as psychoanalysts specialize in longer-term psychodynamic treatments, so feel free to ask about this subspecialization if you intend to engage in a longer-term

RN

Registered nurse. A nurse who has 2–4 years of education and training and is responsible for basic and advanced nursing care.

LPN

Licensed practical nurse. A basic-level nurse who has at least one year of training and has passed a state-administered licensing exam.

Treatment

111

treatment. Psychiatrists, psychologists, and social workers can also specialize in cognitive or behavioral therapies and should be willing to discuss these treatments with you.

Selma's comments:

These options can be helpful in different ways, but your decision would be easier if you seriously considered your goals. Our family practice physician referred me to a psychoanalyst for treatment of my depression and anxiety. I was young and a senior in high school; this provider did not practice in the town where I lived, so there were many logistical problems. Through the remainder of high school, I went to him twice a week, and sometimes four times a week if things were difficult. After I graduated I moved to his town and went two or three times a week for the next few years. This treatment was psychotherapy by a psychiatrist/ psychoanalyst, which is vastly different from psychotherapy with a caretaker who does not have psychoanalytic training. Often I felt his comments and viewpoints were not relevant and made no practical sense. I accused him of thinking only like an analyst, when it seemed to me that a nonanalytic point of view would make more sense. His answer was, "How else would you expect me to think?"

I would leave annoyed and angry, but at the same time, I couldn't get his comments out of my mind. The more I thought about his inane comments, the more a new way of looking at something—previously not even in my realm of already introspective thinking—opened up. I could then never go back to a past view, which became more superficial or irrelevant. I was amazed, at not only how his thoughts fit my dilemmas, but also how they incorporated me. I felt deeply understood in a way that I could not even articulate. There it was, not only a much-appreciated protection of myself, but also a recognition of who I was. I saw that I had hidden myself from my own world and from myself.

In those two years, I married, had a child, and moved away from that city. But then I knew that what I wanted in my life was to have a complete analysis, however long it took and at whatever cost. It became my top priority. I was less concerned that my treater be a psychiatrist, psychologist, social worker, or counselor, however intelligent and understanding, than that he or she be a psychoanalyst. I knew the others couldn't provide me with the search I needed to do and would only lead to time- and money-wasting detours. My depressions had much eased and I was living a constructive, good life. But I knew my propensity for self-destructive behavior. I also knew that many of my problems were generational in nature, and I was determined that my children would have different responses and experiences than I had as a child. I was resolute that certain disastrous relationship patterns from my family of origin would end with my new family. I wanted not only to live a better life than my parents had, but to pass that wish on as well to my own children for their adult experiences. That was my rationalization for the time commitment and the expense.

When I started analysis again, I had four children. I cannot describe the meaning of my analysis to my husband and to my children nor how it changed the structure of their experiences. Of course, my children can never know; their growing up years in no way paralleled my own because of my treatment. What remained true to both of these analysts was their comments and observations remaining so original to me and so different from anything I would have thought of myself. Once I could get over my anger or amazement, these comments brought an insight and awareness, that, once grasped, I could never forget. I developed in myself a feeling of having not only better choices but also a sense of having choices when I previously thought I had none. I became more constructive, creative, and happier when my anxiety lifted. For me, the only choice was treatment with a psychoanalyst.

69. What are the most important things to find out from my doctor when I am figuring out a treatment course?

The most important thing is to figure out how you can be helped. This process starts with proper diagnosis, including an evaluation with a psychiatrist and possibly an internist/general practitioner/family doctor/gynecologist. Once you have received a rough idea of your type of diagnosis, questions of time, money, medication, and therapy all arise. You and your doctor need to determine what kind of treatment might help you and compare this recommendation with what you feel you can do. Keep in mind that few patients want to come in for therapy at the beginning, so it may be important to secure a plan from the start that has a reasonable probability of working and that can be adapted over time to your willingness to engage in treatment.

Separately, you need to discuss time and money. A four-times-a-week psychoanalysis necessarily differs from a monthly psychopharmacology visit. Look at your insurance coverage and see if your provider is in or out of your insurance network. See if you and your provider can make arrangements to set up a treatment frame—e.g., once-a-week treatment with a psychotherapist (psychiatrist, psychologist, social worker, or nurse) with monthly visits to see a psychopharmacologist as indicated. Once you have a sense of the recommended therapy and a sense of the time and money you are willing to invest, try to put those two parameters together and see what happens. It may be a matter of finding a provider who is in your insurance network or of finding the right fit between you and your provider. Usually any questions regarding publicly available information about the therapist or his or her training are welcome, as should be questions of fees, policies, and work with family members. Think twice if what you hear does not make sense to you; a consultation with a different professional can often make all the difference, even if it confirms that the first treatment provider was on target. Anyone worth his salt welcomes a second opinion.

Selma's comments:

In discussing my treatment, the most important thing was to use my own feelings. This decision would impact a major portion of my life for a long time. Would I be willing to do this, and would I be able? It would mean vacations at a nearby park and resorting to garage sales while our friends furnished their homes, went on trips, and sent their kids to summer camp. I was asking my husband and family to sacrifice a lot for something that only I thought would be infinitely valuable to them. They could not share my treatment with me, and they liked the status quo. Only I knew that what would be better for me would influence the family in healthy, good ways. The children, of course, had no choice; I decided for them much as my friends seriously looked for the best of schools. I wanted the healthiest of mothers for my children. My husband went along with it because it meant so much to me. I had told him when we first met how I felt and I saw the dangers of not working through my longstanding problems. I knew that those 45 minutes a day would likely become the dominant theme of life; I also knew a third

Treatment

115

person would appear in our marriage. I had to make these decisions. And even though I did not discuss my analytic work, its effect was everywhere in new ways. I saw the dynamics of my family change in ways that could not have existed before.

For example, one morning my teenage daughter came into the kitchen in a fury. Nothing was right. Her hair didn't curl, her essay assignment was terrible, and she had argued with her boyfriend and a girlfriend. She took an egg out of the refrigerator and dropped it. I was able to watch her fury without commenting, getting upset, or telling her to calm down. In fact, I was able to stay cheery. She grabbed her books, said goodbye, and started out of the house to school. I replied, "You're going to get your period." She just stared at me, said "No, I am not, it's not due," and stormed out. At three o'clock she called me to pick her up and said, "I got my period. I can't believe you. You're a witch; how did you know?" I said, "You told me when you dropped an egg." We both laugh now about her mother's being a witch.

Had this happened years before between my own parents and me, I know my anger would have stimulated their anger. They would have taken my anger personally, and in minutes we would all have been in a major fight, none of us knowing how the flare-up ever got started. Such harm would be done, especially the separation and isolation that would result from such hostility and defensiveness. The incident with my daughter demonstrated a developing closeness between us that saw us through many difficult later years, which we could not at that time foresee. This closeness grew as a function of the decision I made in asking my family to sacrifice for what became both mine and the greater good—the decision to pursue my treatment.

PSYCHOTHERAPY

70. What are the different kinds of therapies?

In general, you might think of treatment as being split into pharmacotherapy and psychotherapy. The former involves seeing a physician for medication, and the latter is talk therapy. A split treatment involves seeing a therapist for talk therapy and a psychiatrist for medication; a combined treatment means seeing a psychiatrist who can do both (some psychiatrists work exclusively as psychopharmacologists and only see patients for medication work).

Psychotherapy has a seeming infinity of schools of thought, practitioner styles, history, and scientific claims to the "truth." This dizzying array can make it difficult to navigate some of the choices you may face. A few basic parameters can help make sense of the chaos.

Does your therapist believe that unconscious conflicts may contribute to your anxiety? If so, then he or she will likely recommend that you be in some type of "dynamic psychotherapy," meaning that the dynamics (or different feelings, thoughts, and memories that shift in a fluid equilibrium) of your mind might in large part lead to the symptoms from which you seek relief. This kind of therapy can go along with medication, which might also help you free associate, or say whatever it is that comes to your mind, in addition to relieving some acute manifestations of your anxiety. In the most intense form, your therapist might recommend psychoanalysis as a treatment, which would involve meeting four times a week with your analyst to understand in a deeper way

117

what most troubles you and to give you the chance—with the therapist's help—to make better sense of your symptoms, thoughts, feelings, and choices. More frequently, he or she might recommend a once- or twice-weekly therapy, where a basic modification of many of these principles takes place. A psychoanalyst might, relatively, work more quietly, while this kind of therapist might be more active and say more. Any therapist should remain reserved and neutral enough that you can use this kind of treatment as a laboratory within which to recreate in the therapy the very conflicts that most trouble you in your life outside the therapy.

Dynamic psychotherapy can prove invaluable because it is not session-limited and can engage many aspects of your mental life. You will have a chance to make sense of the meaning your symptoms might have for you in a greater way. For instance, if you fear touching things in general but only get panicky when you touch something that belonged to your father, there will be lots to think about. These treatments can also help you integrate other parts of your life with your symptoms. A phobia that keeps you from traveling will hamper your relationship with your spouse or children; being able to resolve these issues with your treatment makes a lot of sense. A more dynamic type of treatment takes into consideration the totality of your life—its meaning to you and its overall course.

If your therapist does not believe that unconscious conflicts are contributing to your anxiety, or if your therapist acknowledges unconscious conflict as a contributing factor to your symptoms, but believes that your present treatment would be best served by a more limited course at the immediate time, you will likely receive some version of cognitive, behavioral, or time-limited interpersonal therapy. These treatments focus more on the exact symptoms you experience and on their reduction via implementation of a plan, which might involve homework and more active interventions to help you change. After the first 10 to 20 sessions, you and your therapist can make an assessment about the effectiveness of the treatment and where you want it to go. Not uncommonly, patients decide to start a longer term, more dynamic kind of psychotherapy after their symptoms have become less severe. At this point, you may have become more curious about the possible origins of your symptoms than in the immediate need to feel better.

If your life seems to be ripping apart at the seams, your therapist might recommend a more supportive approach. If your panic disorder has left you unable to leave home, work, pay bills, or care for your children in the way you did before, your therapist may ratchet up his involvement with your care, possibly even recommending hospitalization. In addition to discussing the role of medication as a tool, he will work with you on your symptoms and on a plan to put the rest of your life back together. This work will be very active, including the creation of a schedule and a day-by-day plan of attack.

If your symptoms involve your entire family, if your family has suffered with you, or if they have helped enable you to create your symptoms, your therapist might also recommend an augmentation with family or couples therapy. As helpful as addressing the individual links of the chain can be, the only way to study and help the whole system is to bring the whole system under surveillance. Many families have made vast improvements from this work.

If your symptoms might improve by working directly with others who have similar problems, your therapist might also recommend group therapy as an additional modality. Groups have the advantage of conquering the shame that can so often affect people suffering from anxiety. Around the world, twelve-step groups meet to harness the power of the group as a tool to conquer shame and mobilize recovery from all kinds of anxiety. A landmark study by Dr. David Spiegel of Stanford Medical School found that women with breast cancer who received adjunctive group/psychosocial therapy lived twice as long as those receiving no group therapy.[1] Powerful connections are made in these groups, and these connections relieve anxiety.

Selma's comments:

I have friends who see a variety of counselors, usually social workers, for what they deem a small problem in their marriage (generally stated as the other partner's inability to understand their needs). When I ask why not get treatment with an analyst, they say they can handle this struggle themselves, implying that analysis means changing into other than what they are now. As a child, I had an essential sense of myself. It was never articulated, but there was a deep inner feeling that I knew was what I called, "me." I expressed myself in things I liked and things I wanted. Somehow, in my difficult home environment and with subsequent anxieties—especially around separations, like in my stormy adolescence—that sense of "me" disappeared. It no longer existed, without even a memory of the girl I once was.

Some years into my analysis, I was walking on a beautiful spring day, loving the beauty of the world. I realized that for an ephemeral few minutes, I looked at the scene and felt it as I had felt it as a child. Rather than "think" this sense, (like telling myself, "I felt this way as a child") this refound feeling felt different. That feeling I had had long ago of having my own private domain became mine again. Now I am a mature, developed person, but the essential person I was and that I knew to be me, articulated to no one, is again intact. Analysis had in fact changed me. I again had the freedom to be myself and to move away from all the defenses I had built and used in order to cope with my anxiety. I again laid claim to being true to myself. For me, it was analysis that worked.

My treatment was hard work. No one does it except you, yourself. My analyst became a trusted guide, and I suppose the work provided tools to better handle life. But the commitment to hang in there must remain, especially when you hate your analyst, when you are so exhausted from the work that you want only to sleep, and when it seems as if nothing is happening. And when things are happening, because they are happening and because you are changing, you might become very anxious over just about everything. It is hard, slow work, and the benefits are lifesaving and life-giving. Or so it was for me.

71. How does psychotherapy work? Does it work?

If you read about any psychiatric medication, you will learn that most are "mechanisms of action unknown." The same holds true for psychotherapy, making us wrestle in detail with what also makes common sense. Some excellent studies have been published, showing the efficacy of a type of psychotherapy for a particular disorder over a particular time frame, but this work still cannot explain how healing takes place. Dr. Susan Vaughan's *The Talking Cure* does a remarkable job of making the case for psychotherapy's actually changing brain chemistry.[2] She outlines a schema that, if true, would offer one explanation behind a clinical truth that many of us see daily: people get better when engaged in psychotherapy with a therapist whom they feel understands them. Drs. Jerome and Julia Franks' *Persuasion and Healing* takes a comprehensive look at the literature on outcome research and mechanisms of action in psychotherapy.[3] They conclude that in all of the work that has been done, no one has ever been able to show definitively that one form of therapy works better than another. Psychotherapy is extraordinarily complicated, with many interpersonal factors at play. This dynamic of a situation makes it difficult to determine through the scientific method how any given individual might get better when the larger group is studied.

Many of us would say that it boils down to several key ingredients. The first would be the relationship between you and your therapist. While any number of providers might be a "right enough" fit for you, it is important that the fit be right enough. That fit is often easier to feel if the person is well trained, as patients who feel that their therapist is likable but does not know enough seldom stay in therapy. Patients do not improve simply by following a manual (as helpful as a manual or workbook can be) in the same way that they do with a manual and a person whom they feel they can trust and who knows what he or she is doing. In most treatments, you will identify with aspects of the personality of your therapist and perhaps incorporate them into your own personality, whether you are aware of it at the time, or not. Your therapist will have to use his or her personality and life history to make sense of yours, and a human bond has to form in order for this action to take place; this bond provides an essential ingredient in creating the foundation for your recovery. After the bond has formed, you might say that your therapy has worked because it helped you to make your unconscious conscious, to find better compromises to deal with your life's predicaments, to relieve the shame that binds you, to feel less alone, to experience more love, to discover greater intimacies, to wash your hands less often, to speak in public more convincingly, to abuse alcohol less, to earn more money, to love your spouse more, to be a better parent, to tolerate the loneliness and void of your existence better, to feel fewer bodily aches and pains from anxiety, or to just do it all without the need for panic attacks! You are in the land of "mechanism of action unknown." It makes sense that if therapy did not work, people would not go, nor would therapists devote their lives and careers to helping others via the use of this medium.

Selma's comments:

After I left my 45-minute session, I would be in one of a variety of moods. However different these moods, there was no question I was having a strong reaction to the session. There was no way to compare it to, say, a 45-minute class.

Sometimes I left having a laugh at some delicious piece of humor that had been spoken that might not have made sense to another. Or, I could feel elated or understood. I could leave feeling just as much misunderstood, or terribly hungry, or exhausted, or tired and irritable. I could leave with a feeling of awe or excitement, or with profound depression and tears. Whatever it was, there was always much feeling and response to the session. One day I left in deep thought; I was on foot and needed to walk to the bus stop. I was so preoccupied and pensive that I just walked by instinct. I crossed a street in the middle of a block, and a cop stopped me for jaywalking. He brought me to attention, as I had been so unaware. I had to go to traffic school to avoid a ticket!

This example became a metaphor for my life. I felt I had been jaywalking all of my life, not being very aware. I had gone in some strange zigzag (that could be dangerous and disastrous) and moved along by instinct to avoid being hit or killed. The cop came to symbolize my analyst, and the traffic school represented my analysis, a place where I became aware of the dangers I put myself in. I learned of the people who would suffer terribly as a consequence of my being hurt or killed and who loved me (my family). I saw I could live a better life going by the rules. Crossing with the lights at the corner meant knowing where I was going and with a good sense of direction.

Another time, I was very discouraged and angry with myself. I felt extremely anxious that past repetitive, destructive behavior just kept coming up in my life. I felt like the mythological creature whose head you chopped off only to discover more heads appearing in its place. I felt defeated and said this to my analyst. "Why do I do this treatment? I keep at it so long and no changes whatever are happening!" I said this as I arose to leave, and I looked at him.

He just shook his head from side to side. He said quietly, "Oh, my, my, my . . . there are many changes." I walked out and thought about it over that day, night, and weekend. He was right. How could I have said that to him? I was so moved I was close to tears. I had been so critical and unappreciative. Elizabeth Barrett Browning's poem, "How Do I Love Thee?" came to mind, but with reference to myself. Here was the beginning of a love for myself. I became able to count the ways there were changes, and I began to do things and live in ways that gave me a feeling of pride in myself. I could not even remember having this sense of myself before, given my constant self-criticism. I think the excitement and pride I felt, but had not allowed myself to feel because of this deep anxiety, maybe matched how I must have felt when I took my first steps as a baby. But there was a difference. When my own children started to walk, my mother would smile but then gasp, "Oh, oh," and run after the baby to grab her. I asked, "Why do you do that?" She told me she was afraid the baby would fall and that she wanted to prevent her from falling. I was then in analysis, and I could realize then that undoubtedly she had done that with me, and I not only became fearful of the consequences of walking, but could see for myself that her fear of my developing separate abilities instilled a deep fear in her that was transmitted to me to as a toddler. I became fearful of every step I took that implied separation, long after I was no longer a child. I was learning to walk again through the analysis, and this time with encouragement. I could not understand what that meant until I went through it myself.

72. How important is the way I feel with and about my doctor?

Your feelings with and about your doctor are absolutely critical. The person who treats you will be responsible for creating a safe, therapeutic environment and relationship in which and with which to heal. In order for recovery to start, it is important that you feel as comfortable as possible in the frank discussion of painful, at times traumatic, parts of your life history and symptom course. The gut feeling you have about the person administering your treatment cannot be overstated. You are entrusting your mind and health care to this person, and choosing

Treatment

well can, in the long run, save a lot of problems, time, and money. Many aspects of the psychotherapeutic treatment involve the therapist's personality as much as what he or she may know, so it is important that this fit be good enough for you to get better.

Having a good feeling about your therapist does not mean, necessarily, liking your therapist, especially as the work deepens. In particular, if you work more deeply to understand painful, difficult aspects of your personality, the therapist may eventually and predictably assume roles of significant people from your past, not all of whom were likable (if one of your symptoms is anxiety). This phenomenon is called transference, and it can be of high yield in illuminating patterns that you bring to the table time and again in your expectation of an anxiety-provoking situation. Feeling that your therapist is about to beat you or trigger explosive feelings of rage does not stir warm feelings and affection. In contrast, overliking or idealizing your therapist can be just as useful in learning about situations that you might find disturbing. To flip the transference example around, you might find yourself thinking your therapist is one of the neatest, most intelligent, likable, warm people you have ever had the good fortune to meet, feelings which in aggregate can help hide deeper fears of being taken advantage of, hated, or abandoned.

No matter whether your therapist takes on a likable or unlikable role, any good therapist conveys a sense of seriousness for the work at hand and respect for your life history as an individual. This sense of safety can be felt and appreciated, even if you hate your therapist in the moment. With a skilled therapist, these feelings of hatred can be understood as important communications in conjunction with what you have been working on recently. This interface illustrates the value of competence. An experienced therapist can help the patient learn the real value of making sense of the feelings he or she has in any moment. These exchanges transcend the patient's need to like the therapist, or the therapist's need or wish to be liked by the patient.

Selma's comments:

The years that I was in analysis, I was heavily involved in the arts. I was an actress, on stage a lot, and very much a part of the city's arts community. I attended opera, dance, and music performances. Our city is not large, and my analyst was also a music and opera aficionado, so our paths crossed frequently. One time he told me he was at a high school music evening and saw my daughter on the dance team. I said, "How did you know my daughter?" (The dance team had well over 30 girls, all dressed identically; in my opinion, they all looked alarmingly alike.) He said, "She looks just like you."

I thought about that comment a lot. For a man who didn't say much, this came as a surprise. He, however, was on my mind night and day. I didn't think he ever thought of me. Besides, I had great worries that my constant repetitive complaints must bore him. I realized that he did think of me, and I took comfort in his remark. I was surprised to learn how important it was to me that he ever thought of me. I took the sort of comfort one feels when they find they have a friend whom they didn't know about.

One night after a performance of a play I was in, I checked the house tickets and discovered that he had come to the play with his wife and had sat way in the back. In our next session, I thanked him, being so surprised and pleased that he had attended. (He certainly knew the agonies I had endured in its preparation.) I told him that I could have found him

Treatment

tickets up front, but he said only that he preferred to sit in the back. But I derived the same pleasure I had before from the high school performance comment. I was making myself very vulnerable in this analysis, and I had a lot of emotion about all of this. It was a comfort to know that this quiet, impassive-looking person had a response to me and actually did think about me. It came as a revelation, and a nice one.

Another time I received a bad review and was angry and hurt. I was playing a prostitute in a comedy, which the reviewer had found to be too realistic and harsh, he wrote, for a comedy. I complained about this in analysis. First, my analyst said he thought the reviewer was upset by his own feelings to such a realistic portrayal of this character. But really, as it was a comedy, why did I not smile? He had noticed it too, as he had seen the performance. The wealth of material and work we did just on this comment made all the weeks of rehearsal and all of the other work so worthwhile. It was phenomenal.

I had monumental work to do, and it absolutely could never have been done if I had not been able to care about my analyst. It was not a business relationship, and it was not a technical one. He was my well-trained doctor and unusual kind of friend in this enterprise toward which we both gave time, respect, thought, and hard work. We made ourselves open and trusting to one another. He occupies a place in my life that is unique, and without love, affection, and respect, it could never have happened.

73. What are signs that a therapist might be inappropriate?

As in the answer to question 72, the most important sign would be your gut feeling. If you have a sense of the creeps around the professional evaluating you, pay attention. If this feeling cannot be explored with the therapist in a way that leads to productive and useful understanding of your life's story, then you're probably with the wrong person. Even in the best of hands, there are times that for reasons unclear to us, the fit simply may be off. You will be better served by taking care of yourself and finding a treatment provider with whom you feel more comfortable.

Other behaviors that would concern me include, but need not be limited to, any therapist who would wish to extend the professional relationship to a personal one; chronically run late; speak at length about his or her personal life or other patients he has treated in more than a brief, situational way for purposes of education; lose her temper with you or speak judgmentally about your actions other than in an attempt to keep the treatment and/or your life safe; prove unable to listen genuinely to your anger with him or her and take that communication seriously; attempt to introduce you to fellow patients in his or her practice; seek advice from you in your own field or specialty; or treat your case history as less than confidential. Any professional who would wish to date you or involve sexual practice as a component of the treatment would be predatory, abusive, and in violation of the law. If this occurs, you are being abused, not treated. Getting the appropriate help means leaving that relationship and considering the impact of what has happened with someone expert in the realm of boundary violations. You might start the process of finding a clinician with experience in these matters by contacting the director or the ethics chairman of your local American Psychiatric Association or American Psychoanalytic Association branch.

If you believe that your therapist has been inappropriate with you, you deserve a second opinion. Obtaining

Treatment

this evaluation can serve several functions and often leads to a positive outcome. You might learn that, in fact, your therapist has been inappropriate by taking advantage of you or by working countertherapeutically with you. A second opinion might provide the catalyst you need to arrange for a safer, more therapeutic treatment. A second opinion might also help you to understand any distortions you may have added to your own story of what felt so inappropriate at the time but in retrospect seem more like overreactions. The consultation with a neutral party in these examples honors the tradition of all good psychotherapy—that speaking openly and on the record about your mind's experience and your actions can yield relief from the very underlying anxiety that can create distortions so powerful that we might believe our therapist wishes to abuse us. In this spirit, the consultation can facilitate a safe return to the prior treatment and psychotherapist.

Twelve-step groups work via a different model—using the full strength of the group—and may be much more social than an individual treatment. Commonly, there is less of a boundary between group leader and group member, as often self-revelation on behalf of the leader allows the group to stand justly on even ground. Such revelation is thus entirely appropriate.

74. How important is my actual diagnosis in determining the kind of treatment I get for myself?

Your diagnosis is crucial. As illustrated in various vignettes throughout the Faces of Anxiety section, we make mistakes when we do not make the right diagnosis. While it may take several months or years to know with certainty what any given individual's diagnosis may or may not be, it is always important to rule out the most severe diagnoses. This process usually begins with a careful medical workup, perhaps including a trip to the neurologist for an **EEG** or a CT scan of the head. It always begins with a detailed, careful life and psychiatric history. If your doctor believes that you suffer primarily from an anxiety disorder, he or she will have ruled out depression, manic depression, and substance abuse diagnoses as primary. If you are solidly within the anxiety spectrum, then it may be less important to determine if you have pure panic disorder, social phobia, or both, for example. You will have a chance in your treatment to discern what most troubles you, the ways in which it appears, and whether you would be willing to consider the use of medication as a tool to manage your symptoms.

If you clearly have obsessive compulsive disorder (OCD) or panic disorder with agoraphobia, the diagnosis helps your doctor to know that you would most likely benefit from a trial of medication and some version of cognitive, behavioral, and exposure therapy. If you clearly have posttraumatic stress disorder, then you will most benefit if in treatment with someone experienced in that field. Otherwise, you can refine your diagnosis as treatment unfolds. Most patients do not fit neatly into the boxes of the DSM and suffer from an overlap of symptoms. Finding a treatment that places the focus on you as an individual and your life history and symptoms rather than on your diagnosis per se will allow for the real story, whatever it might be, to unfold safely.

EEG

Electroencephalogram. This is a kind of brain imaging technique, involving electrodes placed around the scalp, that measures brain waves and can detect abnormalities like seizures.

Treatment

131

Rick's comments:

While I have a long-term diagnosis of depression, it is relatively recently that I have been diagnosed as having OCD. This is not the fault of any of the people I have seen in treatment. My OCD mostly takes place internally, with thoughts that hinder me, yet are not really observable to others. My clinical workers are not psychic, and since I found it very difficult and embarrassing to talk about the nonsense phrases, word and number avoidances, and repetitive thoughts whose origins I either can't explain or wouldn't want to, I was not considered to have this illness until I began to talk openly about these symptoms. I am currently looking to find a psychiatrist in my neighborhood with whom I can work by taking medication and participating in talk therapy, in addition to seeing my current therapist.

I would urge anyone who is reading this and is not getting the help that they need—and deserve!—because of any misguided shame they may be feeling about the nature of their symptoms: don't lose valuable time the way I did by concealing things a clinician can aid you with. There is nothing "bad" or "silly" about what you are dealing with. There are reasons OCD occurs and there are ways OCD can be treated. There is no reason that that treatment can't begin soon, or now.

75. Why is being listened to and feeling understood so important to any good treatment?

Patients do not return to see us because of our choice of medication or because of our ability to make a correct diagnosis quickly, though those aspects of care may factor significantly into that decision. Patients return because they feel listened to and taken seriously. A patient may kick and scream, tell us how much they hate us and how unsafe they feel in our hands, only to sign up immediately when a regular hour opens. Patients vote with their feet rather than their words. Feeling truly understood by another individual with your most honest feelings—comfortable or uncomfortable—is perhaps the most powerful force between humans, and that feeling may well draw on the healthiest aspects of early mother-infant interaction. As humans, we crave to be understood, and finding a doctor or therapist who makes you feel understood is essential. If you know that your doctor takes you and your story seriously, then you can feel comfortable delaying the need for a diagnosis until your doctor has the data she needs to make one correctly, even if that takes a couple of years working closely with her and allowing her to experience with you the ups and downs of your particular life.

Finally, being listened to and taken seriously in and of itself reduces anxiety. Knowing that there is a person and a place to help contain and understand your feelings makes the feelings more manageable. Learning to understand the origins of these feelings can only occur with someone who listens to you closely enough to understand some aspect of what you go through. Good listening is the flip side of the talking cure coin.

Selma's comments:

"If I had 100 tongues in my head, I couldn't completely tell you all the thoughts I have nor the different attitudes I have to those thoughts," I said to my analyst. I didn't know where to start or what topic to choose. So I started with the one that just seemed to need to be spoken the most, without knowing the certain digressions I would make or where I would end up with this free association process. I can be pretty funny, or

quite down on myself, or very dramatic. In truth, I used a good deal of these styles convincingly to deflect what I really felt at the time. Growing up with very needy, unhappy parents, I had become competent and sophisticated in smoothing over any rough material. It became my second nature to push away growing, gnawing, upsetting thought patterns which brought on anxiety. I didn't even have to plan it, as my thinking style just dealt with anxiety that way.

Somehow my analyst listened carefully for the main thread of what I tried to say but which at the same time got negated or circumvented. He listened for my need or the feeling in the moment. I was never too aware of this, as I kept talking and would get caught up in the immediacy of my thoughts. Then he might say something, something I might think was off the wall. Or, maybe he would hit home, leaving me feeling deeply understood in a way I didn't realize even existed. I was not sure if he was using some kind of magical insight, or maybe it was that he was picking up on something in my tone of voice that shocked me. How could he have heard that, when, surely, that couldn't possibly have come from any message of my own.

But one way or another, we have moved to a different position and to another viewpoint that has a lot of meaning for me, whether I can accept it at the moment or not. And my life has changed; I can't go back. And there it is. If he were to listen as my good friends do on the phone or at a party, or even as a best friend might listen, this change would not happen. In those circumstances I might feel vastly better through the socialization with people I know and like. But I would not have changed in the same way.

The analysis moves forward because the analyst listens. No listening, no development. Maybe this is one way for you to check if yours is the right health-care provider. If nothing happens, maybe you are not being heard. I was.

76. What do I do if my time and/or money are limited?

The managed care era has borne witness to a conscious, calculated attempt to reduce costs of health care. The complexity of the mind and its symptoms over the course of a human life do not fit neatly into the cost-saving clinical algorithms used to determine medical necessity in mental health treatment. Some companies respond with impossible bureaucratic obstacles, making reimbursement for services far more difficult than before. Some will only allow reimbursement with an unprecedented intrusion into the confidentiality of the doctor–patient relationship. Do not be surprised to find yourself with inadequate psychotherapy or substance abuse treatment benefits relative to the need of your condition. Managed care companies prefer psychopharmacologic treatment models that focus on prescription medication and the use of a psychiatrist primarily as a dispenser of medications; these models cost less money. Psychotherapy, particularly good psychotherapy with a trained professional, can cost significantly more money. Furthermore, many psychiatry residency training programs across the country no longer teach dynamic psychotherapy to their psychiatrists in training; in this way the residents can see many more patients per hour and week, thus providing care for more at less additional cost.

Patients often end up with insufficient resources, particularly if they have no health insurance. When this

Treatment

135

becomes the case, one option involves looking into treatment options at either academic medical centers, public hospitals and clinics, or through psychoanalytic institutes' treatment clinics. Departments of psychiatry, which run mental hygiene clinics staffed by residents, may offer treatment at a lower cost, while the residents receive supervision from more senior staff. What residents lack in gray hair or sophistication is usually offset by their enthusiasm, interest in patient care, and openness to the treatment relationship. Resistance to treatment exists at all levels; as one apocryphal supervisor said, "when I was young, people complained that I was too young and inexperienced to treat them, and when I became old, they told me I was too out of touch to treat them." Psychoanalytic institutes also often offer psychotherapy and psychoanalysis at a reduced cost with their members in training. To find an institute near you, you can log on to *www.apsa.org* and go from there.

Selma's comments:

Time

My life for decades revolved around the 45-minute hour I spent from Monday through Friday in that darkened library/office with that couch. I was very active in community life, often centered (but not wholly) on my children and husband. I was hugely involved in theater, where I acted, took workshops, and taught acting and drama. Frequently I had paid jobs, such as project director for an organization. I always took classes of some kind and did hosts of committed volunteer work. In other words, I did not live a passive, withdrawn life, even though there were times that I considered myself to be that when I left the analytic hour. The view others had of me seemed to be vastly different. I didn't consider myself any dif-

ferent than I was before I had started this treatment, and I didn't consider myself to be very different from my friends.

Respect was perhaps the greatest attitude I learned in analysis. My parents never respected me. They passed over respect, as it seemed to be unnecessary. After all, I was a child. My analyst respected my feelings and me; I had never had that before. Respect was new for me, and it took a long time for me to believe it and to understand it. But once that happened, it was like lifeblood. I did not discuss with anyone where I was from 10 to 11, or whatever the hour was. I was afraid that if I shared my newfound knowledge with everyone, I would lose it. That is, I would make myself lose it. I did not believe I would be able to tolerate the jealousy I imagined others would have and would soon give it up. So I kept it all private so that I could keep it. I became very clever about arranging my schedule so that I could disappear for an hour a day. And I did. Many times the commitments I had and what I had to do to change my schedule became a strain and irritation. But there was never any doubt in my mind about what I was going to go. I was going to my treatment. There was no bond in my life as strong as that bond. And I don't know why, but I would be there, day after day. The thought that it was difficult was not on my mind. Sometimes the time there was painful. Maybe I couldn't talk, and maybe I could only whimper with a knot in my throat. But skip it? Never.

Money

The words I dreaded to hear from my analyst were, "I will have to raise my fee." Maybe he also said, "I am sorry . . ." but I have blocked out that memory. It didn't happen too often, but I went for many years; and it was announced now and again. Fees were never lowered. I always accepted this reality, and I never commented, even though I was always angry and hurt. I shared so much with him, and in my free association talk, he learned of the struggles we had with five children, a salaried husband, and the financial commitment I had given myself with the analysis. He seemed to have no compassion for that. I went through depressions over this, and in the end, I always accepted it. We made other concessions in our lives to meet this need. The alternatives—to cut down on my hours, or to end them—were unacceptable to me. I suppose I could have discussed the fee with him, but I never did. Even being in analysis, one doesn't actually become what one is not. I suppose the fear of separation was too strong in me to threaten what I would see as rupturing this relationship.

I found my rationalization for the acceptance, and they were pretty good rationalizations. Our oldest girl was then in college. She came home to visit and told us that her professor in the first lecture of the school year said that if, at the end of four years, she and her fellow students still admired their parents, then the school would have failed. She came home to tell us that she loved us and wanted to see us, but that we had to keep these visits secret so that she did not fall out of favor with her friends. Rough times were ahead; our children were growing up, and life could be harsh, not what we had hoped it to be for them. I was not only able to hold it together for myself, but also able to keep the strength of our family's ability to communicate intact and to help each other during stressful times. I was still in analysis, and it proved worth everything I had invested in it. I had made good decisions with my life. We drove second-hand cars and still had no bedroom set. But the important things, like love and understanding in our family, were stronger than ever and still growing, even though life was now more complicated with grown children, their spouses, and grandchildren. I have never been sorry for the expense but rather consider myself lucky to have been able to have afforded this chance to rearrange formerly self-destructive patterns from my childhood. Today, the cost seems immaterial. But it would be untruthful to say that it didn't matter. It did, and I had a lot of feelings about it. I also made the right decision.

77. What is cognitive behavioral treatment?

Cognitive behavioral treatment (CBT) is a rubric that, loosely defined, attempts to treat different mental health struggles via a systematic examination of the cognitive and the behavioral aspects of any particular disorder. In the example of panic attacks associated with flying, various distortions in thinking occur while numerous distortions of behavior can occur. CBT assesses these directly with the patient in 10 to 12 sessions, often using a homework-style approach. The results can be remarkable, as the patient learns to break down the various components of his anxiety and thus becomes more in control of it. A patient's thinking distortions would include thoughts that the plane will likely crash or that he would likely die from a panic attack while flying. Reassuring the patient against their feared likelihood of a crash or heart attack versus the reported statistics can begin to address these themes. Addressing the behavioral avoidance of the airport and air travel by creating a plan to desensitize the patient gradually to the idea of air travel, traveling to the airport, and in time, purchasing and taking a trip can help the patient regain confidence. At the same time, you simulate fast heart rate, shortness of breath, and dizziness by recreating those symptoms in the office and teach the patient that they learn to reassure themselves when symptomatic. Active exposure to the panic-inducing situation is elemental to the treatment, as is detailed record-keeping of different physical symptoms and thoughts, with or without combined medication. CBT can be very effective in helping

CBT

Cognitive *behavioral* treatment. A form of psychotherapy that has been proven to be particularly helpful in anxiety and depression.

Treatment

139

a patient quickly gain control over what otherwise had been crippling symptoms.

78. What do I do if I start to develop anxiety about my treatment and/or my doctor?

Patients commonly experience anxiety about their treatments. These reasons range from reality to manifestations of the patient's anxiety.

Some of these issues have been addressed earlier (see question 73, regarding inappropriateness of the therapist). However, even with an entirely appropriate therapist, anxiety can emerge as a function of the treatment. This anxiety can be very painful and uncomfortable, and one of the easiest ways for the mind to trick itself is to attribute the cause of the discomfort to the therapist. One of the most common examples involves the increased closeness of the therapist and the patient. As patients begin to discuss their lives and their symptoms, it becomes clear why they may not feel safe in the world, or they may come to expect that the same traumas that have occurred before will happen again, this time in the room with their therapist. Patients commonly become concerned that the therapist will control them with medications, make their sexual orientation homosexual, exploit their financial resources, or take advantage of special professional information (e.g., stock tips). These, as general examples, show a fear of trusting the therapist. It can be so much easier for the patient to believe that the therapist is untrustworthy or less than ideal than it is to believe that he has experienced again the same fears of closeness that he lives with in his relationships outside of the therapist's office. With any good therapist who understands a patient's need to recreate in the room the very patterns that frame that patient's thinking and feeling outside of the room, these anxieties can usually be understood as important markers in the patient's treatment course. If your therapist does not seem to feel comfortable discussing your anxieties, either about the therapist or anything else, then you might wish to seek a consultation with someone more experienced.

Selma's comments:

Slow, slow, slow. There were times, too many it seems, that it felt as if there were never going to be change. I would say to myself that this treatment was a waste of money. I had subjected my family to privation for what? I was the same, indeed, it seemed to me, if not worse. My former glowing self image of my astounding the world with my great acting talent, or of receiving kudos over a brilliant piece of writing were not happening. Instead, I was living over and again the destructive relationships I spent hours on the couch saying that I understood in lucid, articulate terms. My eating habits that had caused me such agony refused to budge; my hypersensitivity to a 1-pound weight gain still kept me home mortified.

Why was I wasting this time and money? Better it should go to someone who could apply him- or herself better. I saw it as wasted on me. I remember telling my analyst once (although not the only time, by any means), that there was no change and that I couldn't seem to get it. I felt I was too dumb. I was literally the dumb blonde I so successfully played on stage. He had no explanations to give me, and he wasn't the vocal type anyhow. I left crying at my failures. But as always, what he said, even though via such minimal statements, stuck with me. In spite of my doubt and agony, I wondered what he

Treatment

meant. Where was there change? I thought his words through. It wasn't the kind of change to write a book about.

With much difficulty, I had seemingly automatically responded differently to those relationships within which I now had a glimmer of freedom to act differently. And when I wanted to withdraw and to feel sorry for myself, I did at least move and did get out of the house. Maybe late, but I got there and got involved in what was going on. These small vestiges of self-respect started to occur. No money could ever rival the value this had for me in starting to take charge of my life. I was beginning to live life with less anxiety.

79. When should I strongly consider the use of medications in my treatment?

The use of medication is always an option for someone symptomatic enough to seek mental health treatment. Several factors guide this decision, the first being the patient's willingness to consider its use. Some patients will simply be too reluctant to consider medication for fear of side effects or fear of the loss of control that they perceive will occur from taking a pill that works on their mind. While these fears may make emotional sense to the anxious mind, and while an excess of any medication that works on the brain could create varying degrees of mental status changes, the primary goal of any carefully tailored medication regime is to gain *more* control over symptoms and unwelcome thinking patterns—or to have all of the desired effects without any of the side effects. Most patients, if uncomfortable enough with their symptoms and, in time, trusting enough of their doctor, will consider the use of a medication if they believe it might help lessen their distress. If you still are too scared to take a medication, do not panic; you are a perfect candidate for psychotherapy with a doctor who specializes in the talking cure.

Most patients have an internal threshold they live with. Something in their lives has tripped a circuit, putting them above that threshold and prompting them to go to a therapist for consultation. If you feel so overwhelmed that waiting to speak with someone feels like agony, you should probably be on medication. If your panic attacks are occurring regularly, if you cannot fly or leave your home, if your ability to work or take care of your family has become impaired, if your ability to read or concentrate has diminished, or if the feeling is one that your internal home has caught fire, then you should probably be on medication. Many pharmacologic strategies are shorter term, so trying a medicine does not have to mean months and months depending on a pill. It does mean making a commitment to feeling better and taking the leap of faith that your doctor will help you find a medicine that works for you. You and your doctor should be able to speak frankly about the risks and benefits of both taking medicine and not taking medicine, so as to help you make more of a free and informed decision.

80. What are the most common types of medications used to treat anxiety disorders, and what would the best kind be for me?

Please see Table 3 for an overview of common medications for treating anxiety disorders. The main idea is to use a medicine tailored to your condition. If you have an accompanying depressive or manic-depressive picture, your doctor would address those conditions as well and strategize with you to use as few medications

Table 3.   Major Medications Used in the Treatment of Anxiety Disorders.

Category	How do these work?	Common examples	Typical dosages	Side effects (of class)
Benzodiazepines	Immediately, on same part of brain as alcohol Create immediate relief	Lorazepam (Ativan) Clonazepam (Klonopin) Alprazolam (Xanax)	1–2 mg up to 3×/day 0.5–1 mg 2×/day 0.5 mg 3×/day	Sedation Addictive potential Physiologic dependence Confusion Clumsiness Withdrawal reaction
Serotonin uptake inhibitor (SRI)	Over several weeks, this class of medicines increases the levels of serotonin in key areas of the anxiety system, creating a gradual dissipation of anxiety.	Escitalopram (Lexapro) Citalopram (Celexa) Sertraline (Zoloft) Fluoxetine (Prozac) Luvoxamine (Luvox) Paroxetine (Paxil)	10–20 mg/day 10–80 mg/day 50–200 mg/day 10–80 mg/day 50–400 mg/day 10–80 mg/day	Sedation Nausea, diarrhea Weight gain Loss of libido Lack of orgasm/ ejaculatory delay Flip into mania/ hypomania
Atypical antipsychotics	In lower dosages, this class of medicines can target symptoms that stem from thinking or mood disturbances.	Olanzapine (Zyprexa) Risperidone (Risperdal) Ziprasidone (Geodon) Quetiapine (Seroquel)	1.25–30 mg/day 0.25–4 mg/day 10–160 mg/day 25–800 mg/day	Weight gain (variable) Sedation Confusion

Table 3. (continued)

Category	How do these work?	Common examples	Typical dosages	Side effects (of class)
Mood stabilizer	Usually effective also in the treatment of some seizure disorders, these medications act to stabilize the cell membranes in areas related to the creation of anxiety.	Valproic acid (Depakote) Lithium (Eskalith) Carbamazepine (Tegretol) Gabapentin (Neurontin)	125–1250 mg/day 300–1200 mg/day 200–1200 mg/day 300–3600 mg/day	Weight gain (variable) Sedation Medical complications (kidney, blood)
Serotonin Norepinephrine (SnRI) reuptake inhibitor	Same as SRI, with norepinephrine contribution at higher dosages	Venlafaxine (Effexor)	37.5 mg/day 300 mg/day	Same as SRI, with some possibility of blurry vision, constipation, high blood pressure, or urinary retention at higher dosages
Beta blockers	By blocking the receptor that drives the heart, these stop the shaking, sweating, or racing heart.	Propranolol (Inderal) Atenolol (Tenormin)	10–20 mg 1–3×/day 25–50 mg 1–2×/day	Low blood pressure leading to light-headedness; asthmatic worsening with propranolol
Stimulants	Calm the distractability and agitation of attention-deficit/hyperactivity disorder (ADHD).	Amphetamines (Adderall) Methylphenidate (Ritalin)	5–60 mg/day 5–60 mg/day	Racing heart, irritability, tremor, upset stomach, loss of appetite/weight

Treatment

145

as possible. If cost becomes a real issue, you might want to consider medications available generically, such as the tricyclic antidepressants (not featured in the table), which usually cause greater discomfort with their side effects. If you have particular issues with public performance, you might consider a beta blocker. Often two medications will be used together, such as a benzodiazepine and a **Serotonin reuptake inhibitor (SRI)**. I think of the benzodiazepines as garden hoses that can be used to immediately water a garden while I think of the SRIs as longer-term sprinkler systems, with the anxiety disorder being like a drought. You may need to begin the watering immediately while also thinking ahead in terms of drought protection.

SRI

Serotonin reuptake inhibitor. A type of medication that is used to treat depression and anxiety by decreasing the rate at which serotonin is metabolized in the nervous system.

81. What do I need to know about the SRI medications?

The SRI medications serve as mainstays in the pharmacologic treatment of anxiety. They work well, safely, and broadly, and they usually address many underlying or accompanying symptoms of depression that may have stemmed from the anxiety. Most patients are able to experience symptomatic relief with a minimum of side effects, at least initially. The most immediate side effects—like headache, stomach upset, or sedation—are usually transient and manageable with ibuprofen or bismuth subsalicylate. Over the long run, side effects such as weight gain and/or sexual dysfunction may or may not become issues. Many patients do not gain weight for the first six months, if they gain it at all. At that time, the anxiety may be much better managed and responsive to psychotherapeutic intervention. Similarly, many patients will report some kind of sexual dysfunction, but many will not. Patients tell me the most about decreased libido, increased time to achieve orgasm, or inability to achieve orgasm. Depression also causes decreased libido, so many patients simply want to feel better and see if their sexual desire improves as a function of the depression's lifting and wait to assess the potential side effects at that time. Some men already suffer from premature ejaculation, which makes the delayed time to orgasm a welcome side effect. Inability to orgasm as a function of the medication breaks the deal for most patients. Thankfully, there are alternatives that cause less sexual dysfunction but still treat depression.

A unique side effect that can go missed while taking an SRI is the induction of mania or hypomania. Characteristically, patients who have this side effect have a history of major depression and/or manic or hypomanic behavior from prior periods in their lives. The SRI simply elicits the elevated aspect of mood. However, there are patients who start to experience hypomanic signs just from the SRI, often at low doses and within the first week or two. Hypomanic behaviors include not needing to sleep as much, increasing euphoria and/or irritability, and feeling like one's mind is moving more quickly than at baseline (mania is a more severe, longer lasting form of hypomania). A hypomanic person might also feel increasingly creative, sensual, sexual, or bubbly. Most patients with hypomania love it and wonder what the problem would ever be, but those people either do not know or have denied the danger of becoming frankly manic. Mania can endanger one's entire career, marriage, and life via the grandiosity, recklessness, and lack of judgment with which it so often presents. Statistically, most patients receive an SRI from a well-intentioned but busy primary care doctor who prescribes it but cannot see the patient again for several weeks. In that time, the induction of hypomanic behavior can take place and can easily be missed by someone not trained to detect the subtleties of these early shifts.

82. What do I need to know about benzodiazepines?

The benzodiazepines often work like a double-edged sword—highly effective in the right situation but also with hazards of their own. They work rapidly, efficaciously, and with a minimum of side effects if dosed properly. They can take a mind which feels like a hurricane in progress and settle it quickly to feel like a reasonably clear day. Benzodiazepines tend to work less well with time and may require greater dosages to achieve the same effect. Without starting a second medication which can be used more longitudinally and with a greater safety margin. Stopping benzodiazepines can be difficult and can risk creating rebound anxiety. As long as you know about the risks of dependency (it can be hard to get off of them without a careful, willful, downward taper of medication), withdrawal (it can be uncomfortable, if not life threatening, to discontinue them cold turkey), and long-term side effects of regular high-dose usage (like memory impairment), then the benefits can be maximized via judicious therapeutic use. I tend to prefer the longer-acting benzodiazepines, such as clonazepam, as they avoid the more sudden shifts in blood level and the accompanying rebound symptoms of anxiety that can occur. Starting a benzodiazepine immediately for relief at the same time as starting an SRI for longer term irrigation can allow a doctor to begin to wean a patient off of the benzodiazepine in several weeks after the SRI has taken root. This strategy works well and without undue complications most of the time.

83. Are antipsychotics ever used to treat anxiety?

The atypical **antipsychotics** have a unique place in the treatment of anxiety disorders. Most of us would begin with either or both of the above medicines (e.g., a benzodiazepine and an SRI). However, some patients cannot take benzodiazepines because of a history of substance abuse or would prefer not to because of that concern. Other patients experience a level of anxiety that can border on psychosis in its intensity, e.g., the patient who refuses to have surgery to remove a malignant cancer because of an overwhelming fear of surgical complications. Still others have mania or hypomania, which can add rocket fuel to speed the anxiously working mind. Usually these medicines can work well in these situations and require far lower dosages than those needed for management of schizophrenia. Most of the more dangerous side effects of this class of medication occur at higher dosages taken for longer maintenance periods of time, making their usage in the context of anxiety mostly safe.

Antipsychotic
a psychiatric medication that is used to treat psychosis (such as hearing voices or paranoia), as well as severe anxiety.

84. What do I need to know about the mood stabilizers?

The **mood stabilizers** primarily assist with the management of mood. Therefore, should you happen to suffer from some type of mood disorder involving more

Mood stabilizer
a psychiatric medication that is used to balance mood states.

Treatment

149

than just depression and the lower end of mood (i.e., some type or problem with mood swings) that also includes anxious features, one of these might be right for you. The particular details of why to choose one medication over another can be quite complicated and usually involve a detailed conversation with your doctor. Time and again, however, patients present thinking that their problem is simply really bad anxiety—and it is—but have also never been properly diagnosed for their bipolar or bipolar spectrum disorder. In those instances, starting a mood stabilizer can make the ultimate difference in the management of the anxiety.

85. What do I need to know about the beta blockers?

Beta blockers work by blocking the beta receptor of the heart, which drives the heart rate. This mechanism also happens to lower blood pressure, which is the primary reason one might take this class of medicine in the first place. However, for the management of stage fright, public speaking, or performance anxiety (test-taking, for example), the blocking of this beta receptor can prevent the body from kicking into overdrive. This technique will make it less likely for the heart to beat fast, and thereby lessen the sweating, shortness of breath, and nausea that can go along with the immediacy of a panic attack. Regular usage of these medications could theoretically lead to depression, but at the lower frequency and dosages used for this situation, this side effect is uncommon. If you have asthma, then you will want to use a selective beta blocker that will not trigger an asthmatic attack.

86. What do I need to know about the stimulants?

A **stimulant's** ability to calm the anxiety of patients with attention deficit hyperactivity disorder (**ADHD**; with or without the hyperactivity part) presents one of the seeming ironies of modern psychopharmacology. A medicine that would give most of us more energy and help most of us concentrate somewhat better (but at the risk of making us overexcited, tremulous, nauseous, or headachy) can smooth the wrinkles out of the ADHD mind. Many patients will report that their world is distractible, agitated, and hypersensitive to stimuli which can lead them to lose control of their temper. The stimulants are a normal first place to start in the pharmacologic management of ADHD and often bring a type of organizing calm as a result. If you are concerned about ADHD, then you might start by consulting your doctor or reading Hallowell and Ratey's *Driven to Distraction*.[4]

Stimulant
a class of amphetamine-based medications that is used to treat ADHD and can sometimes help with the treatment of depression.

ADHD
Attention deficit/hyperactivity disorder. A psychiatric disorder that involves a spectrum of inattentive symptoms and/or hyperactive symptoms.

87. What is the placebo effect?

For reasons that still boggle both the mind and researchers, the placebo effect is powerful. Perhaps due to the brain's power of pattern recognition and expectancy in a given situation, in this culture we usually link going to a doctor, seeing the white coat, and taking a pill with getting better. Patients who take a sugar pill but expect to get better can actually get better because of the expectation and the cascade of brain chemistry it triggers. And if the notion of taking a pill can lead to actual effects, one wonders how else we might be able to access those effects. In psychiatry, in order to be approved a drug must display a statistically significant effect over the placebo rate of improvement, which is often as high as 40%. This pattern tends to mean at least two things. The first is that if a medication is, in fact, approved under these standards, the odds of its actually working for you are high. But it also means that 40% of patients in control groups get better by taking a sugar pill or enrolling in the trial or as a function of receiving the medical attention of the trial's involvement. The placebo effect can help you to harness all other aspects of your mind beyond medication as you seek to mobilize allies in your treatment of anxiety (see Other/Alternative Treatments for Anxiety).

88. What do I need to know about herbal remedies?

The pharmacologic agents discussed thus far have been from the Western medicine chest, meaning that they have been approved by the U.S. Food and Drug Administration. To have done so, they have passed through various stages of clinical trials and have been shown to be more effective than placebo. Most of the evidence for herbal remedies is anecdotal. Because these herbs do not show scientific effect in controlled trials does not mean that they might not help any given individual. However, it does mean that they could create side effects, either alone or in conjunction with other medicines that you might be taking. Herbal remedies are usually found at health stores or dispensed via traditional Chinese medical practitioners. One step that can definitely help you is to let whoever treats you know what medicines you take so that they might be able to troubleshoot against any known adverse effects. As Eastern medicine becomes more welcome in the U.S., many mainstream academic medical centers have

started alternative medicine centers, which can be resources for up-to-date herbal remedy information.

89. How will I know when it is OK to stop taking medicine or to stop my therapy?

The decision to stop medication and/or therapy usually
occurs as a natural outgrowth of a healthy treatment relationship, and unless the patient decides to leave treatment for her own reasons, the two almost never happen
at the same time. This principle follows basic cognitive
reasoning. If the patient presents for treatment of
symptoms of anxiety at point A, receives medication
and relief at point B, and then wonders about how to
proceed at point C, it makes sense—in the patient's
mind—that relief is associated with medication and
point B. In order to have the same relief without being
on the medicine, a further intervention must occur to
prevent the patient from going back to point A. The
utility of psychotherapy here takes on added meaning—in order to get off of medicine, a patient needs
the structural tools provided by therapy!

Depending on the kind of therapy and the goals of any
given patient, different algorithms might apply. Some
might feel comfortable with a short course of CBT and
a transition back to a life without symptoms via some
better coping tools. Others might become curious
about the origins of their anxieties and wish to use the
opportunity of distress as a springboard to a more introspective psychodynamic therapy. As the written
Chinese character for crisis is a composite of the char-
acters for danger and opportunity, so, too, patients can
make the best of their symptoms and learn maximally
from them. Most studies tend to reinforce the notion

Treatment

that patients only taking medicine do less well than those with combined medication and psychotherapy treatments. These more exploratory treatments might go on for years as one clue leads to another and a patient may continue to benefit from using the treatment as a tool to understand further the patterns in her life that have, in their recreation in the therapy, generated the anxiety she lived with day in and out but now occurs less often.

90. What kind of medication reactions could be serious or lethal?

Concerning the medications used in the treatment of anxiety, there are several absolute red flags that any patient on those medications must know about. Please keep the following in mind:

a. Overdose. If taken in excess—either accidental or intentional—any medication can create serious problems. In particular, however, benzodiazepines, lithium, and tricyclic antidepressants can be lethal. The benzodiazepines can create respiratory depression, particularly if combined with alcohol, and can lead to states of unconsciousness or death. Lithium toxicity can present as confusion, slurring of speech, a staggering gait, or kidney failure before leading to a frank comatose state. The tricyclic antidepressants can cause excess sedation and cardiac abnormalities. All of the above can be lethal in suicide attempts, and patients taking those medications should be carefully monitored if suicidality is in any way part of the picture.

b. Withdrawal. All medications can have serious side effects in withdrawal, including a return of the symptoms which have been under treatment, but some are more risky than others. Benzodiazepine withdrawal is one of the potential true psychiatric emergencies, if for nothing else than the patient's lack of understanding of the seriousness of the physiologic dependency that takes place over time, particularly at higher doses of the medication. Immediate signs of withdrawal (the first 24 hours) tend to include sweating, nausea, racing heart, shortness of breath, tremors, and profound discomfort. If no benzodiazepines are taken to replace the relative state of withdrawal, then the patient can progress to *delirium tremens* (just as with alcohol withdrawal). This condition presents with confusion and fluctuating vital signs, which could then cause a stroke, a heart attack, or a seizure with loss of consciousness. If you are taking benzodiazepines, you should be aware of all of the above and educate yourself with your doctor's help.

c. Other. Unusual side effects can accompany any medication. Olanzapine has been linked with high blood sugar, which can trigger the symptoms of diabetes, including coma, if not treated appropriately. Too many stimulants can worsen someone who also has bipolar disorder or any other tendency to have distortions of thinking. Propranolol can trigger an asthmatic attack in those with a preexisting history of asthma.

OTHER/ALTERNATIVE TREATMENTS FOR ANXIETY

91. What would be considered additional interventions for anxiety disorders?

While you will not read about additional interventions in standard psychiatric texts, many patients over the years report all kinds of interventions they have done for themselves to help manage their anxiety. These are harder to study in a strictly scientific way, but I believe they help as augmentation strategies. Patients suffering from the depths of loneliness have gone to the local pound and found a new dog to help fill this void. Others have used humor to lighten up otherwise dark nights of the soul, either via going to comedy clubs, reading recognized humorous literature, or reconnecting with old friends with senses of humor. Still others have developed an artistic pursuit that has provided an invaluable outlet for their depression, be it sculpture, dance, painting, jewelry design, creative writing, dressmaking, or whatever might help translate internal frustration into an external work of art that expresses those feelings.

Rick's comments:

Humor has been a great coping mechanism for me. I love to listen to comedy as well as to perform and to write it on occasion. It would be nice to think that as I search for further help with my OCD and anxiety that I might be helping others who are going through a difficult time by making them laugh. (Once in a while I tell jokes that don't make people laugh, however I don't think they do any lasting harm!) On the other hand, going to a comedy club, if I'm performing, usually doesn't relieve my anxiety. Standing on a stage, in front of strangers, is not necessarily a good anxiety reducer, yet it's an experience I wouldn't have missed for the world. Some anxiety is worth the price!

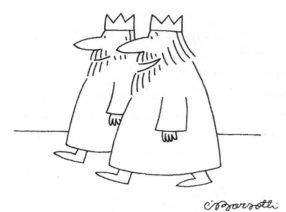

"IT'S AMAZING, SINCE I'VE BEEN TAKING PROZAK THE WHOLE DAMN KINGDOM IS HAPPIER."

Reprinted with permission from The Cartoon Bank, a division of *The New Yorker* magazine.

92. Can I ever get virtual reality treatment or treat myself on the Internet?

These questions raise the possibility of treating oneself. If living abroad in a country where you cannot find a psychiatrist who speaks your language, this becomes an even more relevant question. If you are so phobic and/or scared of doctors that you cannot leave your house or see a doctor as a function of your anxiety, then it also becomes relevant. In short, it is important to do whatever works for you. I am not aware of any Internet-based treatment Web sites, though an abundant number of Web sites exist for you to learn more about anxiety disorders. Because interaction with people is a common fear in anxiety, interaction with a treatment professional can be therapeutic. This factor, in conjunction with taking the step of obtaining the right diagnosis from a professional, makes consultation in person the best starting point. If you are abroad or are attempting to seek help for a relative abroad, or if you are unable to leave home, one place to start is Dr. Edmund Bourne's *Anxiety and Phobia Workbook*.[5] You could combine this work with a telephone consultation with a psychiatrist in the United States until a more longitudinal strategy can be put in place. If you believe that you have OCD and cannot leave home for fear of contagion or other type of exposure, order Dr. Jeffrey Schwartz's *Brain Lock: Free Yourself from Obsessive Compulsive Behavior*.[6] Getting this self-help can help you make it to a psychiatrist's office or emergency room. If you explain this story over the phone to a mental health professional, he will understand that you are doing the best that you can. He will also know that you are capable of doing more under different circumstances.

Dr. Joann Difede of New York Hospital-Cornell has done interesting work using virtual reality to treat terrorism survivors from New York's World Trade Center. By gradually replaying video scenes of the day, from more benign to frankly traumatic—initially without but then with volume—she has provided a unique kind of exposure therapy with some remarkable results.[7] Her work compels us to ask how much technology of this age might be used to tailor treatments that could desensitize patients to traumatic memories. However, this kind of technique, like any other treatment for anxiety, would best be done with a mental health professional who would know how to incorporate this type of work into the overall treatment of any given individual's program.

93. How could hypnosis help me?

Hypnosis has been used over the centuries to mobilize cure. Today we understand much more of the science behind it. Finding a way to access a deep, hyper-focused, partially dissociated trancelike state allows the power of the mind to exert itself. All hypnosis becomes self-hypnosis, mobilizing an individual's ability to hypnotize himself. The results are compelling and powerful. Patients who learn to use self-hypnosis have fewer symptoms of irritable bowel syndrome, require less pain medication in hospitals, and deliver babies without epidural anesthesia. Hypnosis can also serve in the treatment of phobias and posttraumatic stress disorder, allowing one to imagine oneself taking off in an airplane or revisiting traumatic memories in a more controlled setting. Anyone who performs hypnosis regularly—usually psychiatrists or psychologists—can speak to the power of this technique.

94. How could biofeedback or guided imagery help me?

Biofeedback therapy uses a basic mind-body principle to help one regulate oneself. Most treatments utilize some combination of the following ideas. The patient is hooked up to a set of instruments that monitor heart rate, sweating response, breathing, and brain electrical activity. Focusing on images that help to soothe the patient can, in time, lead to a lessening of all of the above parameters. As the patient learns to correlate the decrease in mental functioning and heart rate with a calming of the mind via the imagery, new mental and physiologic responses become available to the patient at a time of stress. Some interventions can lead, over time, to a marked ability to monitor internal physiologic

Biofeedback

a method of monitoring one's physical responses to anxiety-inducing situations and attempting to lower the anxiety by reducing the physical response.

Treatment

states and thus modulate one's internal environment when experiencing an external stressor.

95. Could acupuncture help me?

If everything you have tried has not worked, or if you cannot tolerate the side effects of a medication, or you simply wish to pursue a more natural course of treatment, acupuncture can prove helpful. Whether it works by energizing the body's own endogenous neurotransmitters, or whether it mobilizes the power of the mind over the body, we know that acupuncture can yield formidable results. If patients in China can have open heart surgery using acupuncture alone, it is not in any way out of line to consider the role acupuncture might play in facilitating your own treatment. For further information, see the reference section's acupuncture source.

A more immediate, almost risk-free compromise which might allow you to assess acupuncture's possible viability as a treatment strategy is the use of an Alpha-Stim SCS cranial electrotherapy device. This unit delivers small electrical charges to each of your ear lobes. This waveform normalizes brain electroencephalogram (EEG) activity, smoothing out the peaks and valleys that can go along with a picture of anxiety. Some patients have reported that this device has really helped in the same way some patients with depression have reported that the stimulation from a light box during the winter helps lift their mood.

96. What are the roles of diet, sleep, exercise, and social activity in maintaining my recovery?

Time and again, we forget how elemental basic functions of our body are to our well-being. While it comes as no surprise that regular sleep, a balanced diet, brisk exercise, and social relatedness correlate directly with patients' reports of feeling better, it also comes as no surprise that we often neglect to take care of ourselves in these basic ways. Sometimes the demands of child care, finances, or the workplace make it impossible to sleep more or work less, and the costs of these demands accumulate. Sometimes we want the best of both worlds—to cheat the demands of our body by thinking we do not need to apply the basic laws of human **physiology** to our own situation and yet still feel just as good and productive. Like with the rest of life, being human means that the bottom line of our personal accounting is a human one. Almost everyone feels better when he is rested, well-nourished, and in shape. Simply making interventions in one of the above departments may make it that much easier for you to manage your symptoms or to help make the transition off of the medications you already take for anxiety.

Selma's comments:

I considered myself cool at one time. I was "with it" in the current scene of what everyone was doing. I thought that this was how people saw me. I thought I was so cool because I had overcome emotion and feeling. I didn't seem to be swayed by anything. I looked at those who got emotional or hysterical or intense or passionate, and while I didn't feel dead, I also didn't feel moved and could coolly look at the situation and wonder why they had to make such a fuss. If there was an argument or reasonable difference of opinion, I moved away, and I agreed with everyone. Never did I use the term "anxiety" about myself. I had no anxiety, as I thought I was above the emotional capacity to have it.

At the same time, I was running myself ragged and exhausted. I took care of friends, skipping food for 3 days and

Treatment

Physiology
having to do with normal functioning of body systems and organs.

161

then eating ice cream nonstop, and I constantly recriminated myself for what I said to anyone from the bus driver to friends. I felt a gnawing, shaking, physically ominous feeling of lack of control late at night when my husband would have to work. I never used the word anxiety . . . I was handling my life. I was taking amphetamines (prescribed then for weight control as well as depression . . . now called speed) and it dehydrated me. It made me so physically nervous and jazzed up that I also took sleeping pills to relax and sleep, which didn't work; I had severe insomnia due to night frights. I was dreadfully afraid of the night (a carryover from childhood, but my self-control just didn't work with night fright), and I smoked.

Working with my doctor, I stopped cold turkey. It was over . . . the amphetamines and barbiturates, and I never took them again. Finally, a few years later, I was able to end the smoking, also forever. I had tried my theories of diet, sleep, exercise, and social activity, but for me, my attempts were all backward. My idea before treatment had been to weigh 105 (OK, 104, maybe) and I would handle life because I would be so secure in my achievement and able to be the perfect weight to be accepted. I thought my lack of sleep was a major problem; that exercise could help me; and that the social scene was my ticket to success. It took years for me to see the backwardness of my thinking. When I have figured out the roots of my anxiety, diet, sleep, exercise, and social activity are wonderful parts of life. But they are not my problem solvers. When I solve my problems, these become mine with which to enrich my life.

97. Are there any religious approaches to managing my anxiety?

Religion—in its most quotidian and spiritual aspects—can alleviate anxiety. Over the ages, mankind has used spiritual traditions to cope with the human condition and all of its attendant existential anxieties. This question stimulates more thoughts than answers, but several principles come to mind.

If the shoe fits, wear it. If going to church, connecting to the cultural traditions of your faith, or reading scripture helps you to cope with the pain and anxiety in your life, then do it. If prayer helps you access a deeper side within your mind, do it. Without making any comment about any particular faith or the nature of divinity, it seems safe to say that any process which prompts you towards introspection and relationship with a person, power, or force that you esteem serves a self-soothing function.

One principle receiving much focus in Christianity is that of forgiveness. Dr. Robert Karen's *The Forgiving Self: The Road From Resentment to Connection* looks at the psychological function of forgiveness in its genuine, noncoerced form.[8] He states that forgiveness can represent a way of working through the anger of resentment. This function proves useful for the management of anxiety which stems from unresolved rage: the wrongs done us, and our role in still giving them the power to bother us so much. Learning to forgive can go along with working through and letting go of the raw pain from these wounds.

The Buddhist tradition of **mindfulness** also has great power in the management of anxiety. Dr. Mark Epstein makes this case in *Going to Pieces Without Falling Apart: A Buddhist Perspective On Wholeness*,[9] as does Dr. Jeffrey Brantley in *Calming Your Anxious Mind*.[10] The central notion of mindfulness teaches us to allow and hyperfocus on the idea which makes us most anxious. Rather than fight our anxiety or try to disavow it, we allow it; and as we do so we become able, paradoxically, to create

Treatment

Mindfulness
a state of being aware of all of the details of one's surroundings.

163

a distance between it and ourselves. Thus it becomes less threatening and less disturbing. We begin to develop control over it by letting go of the control. Rather than fight the void you feel in yourself and attempt desperately to fill it, you can allow it and thus soothe yourself the process of allowance. This technique is quite powerful—try it, and if you want to meditate, too, then it is even more likely to serve as yet another weapon in your arsenal to manage your anxiety.

98. Where can I find an anxiety disorders support group, and how could that help me?

Group therapy can provide one of the mainstays in treatment for anxiety disorders, and an anxiety disorder support group can provide an essential touchstone. The easiest place to start this process is the Anxiety Disorders of America Association (ADAA) Web site. You can enter your state and zip code and they will contact you with the closest meeting place. You can meet others who have suffered from anxiety, educate yourself more about anxiety disorders, find a referral for treatment, and learn of different group therapy options. The group modality of treatment can prove invaluable with anxiety disorders. The power of the group and the strength drawn from surrounding yourself with others who suffer from symptoms similar to your own yields a calming, stabilizing presence. This technique can combat the feelings of shame and secrecy that so often go along with anxiety. Believe it or not, you are not alone out there.

Selma's comments:

My anxiety disorders support group was comprised of me and my analyst, and it helped me to transform myself from inappropriate energy wasting and life-destroying anxieties. I came to accept life's realistic anxieties, which can be handled. This allows me to live a life that can be constructive and creative and competent with consistent, applied, hard work. This support group involved both of us concentrating and sifting through a problem and allowing it to be disbursed in a different way. With slow, laborious, dedicated work, my life was changed forever.

This support group of two saved my life, and indeed, gave me life. Whatever support group is used, I would think it cannot be an outside-of-you experience. You have to be the most active member of the support group; as it seems to me, the only person that makes the change develop is oneself. There is no question in my mind that I could not have done it without my analyst. No one else or no other group could possibly have supplied that intense concentration on me, coupled with a depth of knowledge and training.

99. What do I do if all else fails?

If all else fails, two major strategies come to mind. If you have tried various treatments that simply have not worked for one reason or another, it may be that you suffer from an unconscious source of anxiety that, were it conscious and available to the surface of your mind, would be more known and amenable to intervention. In these situations, finding a well-trained psychoanalyst who comes with a highly regarded referral in your area can be invaluable. To find one near you, go the Web site of the American Psychoanalytic Association.[11]

If Western medicine and its medical model has failed you, or you feel unable to settle into any of the more traditional Western treatment frames described in this book, then I would recommend you go East. The Eastern medical model—often integrated with the best of what we know in the West—uses a different framework to diagnose and treat disease. Many patients who cannot become comfortable or find effective therapeutics with the Western model have gone East and had success. Why this phenomenon takes place is complicated and may stem from a genuine recognition of the inseparability of the mind and the body. But if all else has failed, you stand only to gain by consulting with the traditional Chinese medical doctor in your area. If your internist cannot help you find one, then you might try the closest Chinese embassy, cultural center, or language center as a point of departure.

Selma's comments:

Everything failing is a thought that never occurred to me in all the years of my analysis. That is not to say my treatment always looked up, forward, or encouraging. There were dark days, weeks of them . . . especially in my adolescence. There were terrible mood swings and deep regressions with destructive behavior and painful, horrible acting out. There were times I wanted to leave, and my doctor would tell me, "you work so hard to see it, and then you throw it all away."

But I never thought of failure or of turning elsewhere. It was like birth . . . you are here and you learn to walk, to talk, and to live; and if it fails, you're dead. So you just keep on working with the problems of life. That's the way I felt about analysis. It was a total commitment. I had found a way that I could live, and if it wasn't working for me, I just had to keep at it harder and more—never less—and it would work out. When the threads twist, you just have to resign yourself to a slower process of unwinding; the knots will come out, but it takes patience.

In fact, I do believe this attitude is essential for success. Otherwise, if you're going to try intense treatment and "better" hasn't happened in 6 months, then you have set yourself up for failure. Theoretically, I suppose if I had felt my analysts weren't good, I might have changed. But I never would have moved away from psychoanalysis. And I would be very cautious about faulting the analyst . . . not that it can't happen that you have one that is not right for you or that you can't have other reasons to change, but you must always examine your own motives. I have talked to people who tell me they have had analysis, and that it did nothing. Much of the time, I discover what they call analysis, and whom they call an "analyst" is far removed from a clinician with the kind of training I mean.

If I were not to choose analysis, the alternative for me would probably be destructiveness in one form or another. I always chose analysis. That, of course, may not be the rule for everyone, but childhood patterns are repeated, no matter how bad they may be. And if one's background incorporates unhappy family dynamics, they will crop up over and over again without much change unless they are worked through, no matter how much your will is to have it otherwise. And that's where you need the commitment . . . that no matter what it takes . . . you will stick at it and work it through . . . with a determination that this will not fail you, as the past so miserably did. Years of dedicated, applied, painful work with a good, trained analyst, and the reward is personal freedom. You can't get any better than that.

100. Where can I find more information?

See the appendix for a selective listing of publications, resources, and references for further information about anxiety. A trip to your local bookstore's psychology section may lead you to all the reference material you need. Finding a doctor who specializes in anxiety in your community can answer many questions, as can contacting the Department of Psychiatry at your local medical school.

Selma's comments:

When I first saw an analyst at 16 years old, I was convinced that no one but me had the depressive feelings and anxieties that I had. I inhabited a world that somehow had been selected by someone for me, or because of my own failures and inadequacies, was mine in which suffering, pity, and contempt were the reigning powers. Everyone else in the world was blessed with desirability and other attributes I could only jealously fathom. I was filled with self-loathing and isolation.

That actually changed the first time I went to my doctor's office. He told me that I wasn't alone and what I was suffering from, and although at that time not carefully delineated, it was common, not only to kids my age, but to people of all ages, and could be helped enormously. He said it was possible I could eat normally . . . as all I had in the 3 days before I saw him were some saltines and jam (not many), and even though I didn't believe him for a minute, I was desperate and wanted to start. He also said astonishing things about girls and their mothers that piqued me as I intensely loved/hated my mother and felt her terrible problem in life was having an awful daughter like me. I was really hooked on these attractive options, and instantly felt not alone for the first time in over a year.

This analytic world became the passion of my life in some ways. I started to read. Someone named Freud had started it all, so I began with The Interpretation of Dreams. *It is hard to explain the changes that came over me . . . the revelation that I was part of a very large world . . . not only that I wasn't alone, but what was going on in my head was universal. That was the first book and the beginning of a lifetime of reading books about psychoanalysis.*

I began to have a deep understanding of insight, of its value and of its need. I could see how helpful it would be for so many people looking sincerely for answers to myriad problems of life, of self, and of family. If only people were alerted to it if it was available, affordable, accessible, and there was knowledge of it.

In all the years that I was in analysis, it was comforting to me to see the spread into so many areas of Freud's emphasis on the influence of infancy and early childhood on adult life. So wherever I was able (there were many opportunities), as president of the PTA, through the boards I was on, conferences I directed, the synagogue and the church (as I had both), I invited analysts to speak on what was appropriate given the situation, but always dealing with children, family, or inner anxiety. These were always free programs, and the talk was always directed to a community audience and was not professional.

The turnouts were phenomenal. My earlier thoughts on my being unique in my set of problems seemed ludicrous. Everything I had suffered belonged to a never-ending, large world, and people were looking for help and answers. The question/answer periods were enlightening, stimulating, and very touching. The respect between the speaker and the audience members filled me with pride about the analytic world. These were wonderful times.

Then something happened. Probably it was the continuing growth of the managed care phenomena, and cost effectiveness started somehow to be a part of the discussion of life's problems. Insurance companies were directing what they would pay away from insight-oriented therapy to medication and quick diagnosis one could find in a manual that did away with the complexity of the mind and the individual. I can't go into all of these changes. There are many others, but for those who are looking for lasting meaningful change that will give them an opportunity for a life of freedom, creativity, satisfaction and happiness, psychoanalysis still exists and is as vital and significant as always, with competent, caring practitioners and a large following. Whether it is called psychoanalysis or psychotherapy (by an analyst), it offers the route to know more about anxiety than any other way.

There are books, meetings, lectures, a lot of information on how to solve problems, live life, or raise children. In all of these venues there is also participation by an insight-oriented therapist or a psychoanalyst. I think the search is not complete or whole until this, too, is explored and considered. When learning more about anxiety and its cures, it is important to consider the distinction between that which will ease immediate pain (a symptom), that which will offer help directed to a cognitive learning self that may or not be applicable to a symptomatic area but will not hold up in the long run, and that which will bring the structural change so that it is changed forever. This is analytic knowledge, and there are proponents of all of this; I believe good self-education incorporates this analytic insight.

Notes

1. "Therapeutic Support Group: David Spiegel," in Healing and the mind, pp. 157–70.
2. Vaughan S.C. (1997). *The talking cure: The science behind psychotherapy.* New York: GP Putnam's Sons.

3. Frank, J.D., & Frank, J.B. (1991). *Persuasion and healing: A comparative study of psychotherapy* (3rd ed.). Baltimore, MD: Johns Hopkins University Press.

4. Ratey, J., & Hallowell, E. (1994). *Driven to distraction*. New York: Pantheon Books.

5. Bourne, E.J. (2005). *Anxiety and phobia workbook*. Oakland, CA: New Harbinger Publications.

6. Schwartz, J.M., with Beyette, B. (1996). *Brain lock: A four-step self-treatment method to change your brain chemistry*. New York: Regan Books.

7. Difede, J., & Hoffman, H. (2002). Innovative Use of Virtual Reality Technology in the Treatment of PTSD in the Aftermath of September 11. P*sychiatric Services*, 53(9), 1083–1085.

8. Karen, R. *The forgiving self: The road from resentment to connection*. New York: First Anchor Books.

9. Epstein, M. (1998). *Going to pieces without falling apart: A Buddhist perspective on wholeness*. New York: Broadway Books.

10. Brantley, J. (2003). *Calming your anxious mind: How mindfulness and compassion can free you from anxiety, fear, and panic*. Oakland, CA: New Harbinger Publications.

11. APSA Web site. www.apsa.org.

Treatment

Resources

Web-based Resources

HealthyPlace.com
http://www.healthyplace.com

American Psychiatric Association
http://www.psych.org

American Psychoanalytic Association
http://apsa.org

Anxiety Disorders Association of America
http://www.adaa.org

Books

Albom, M. (1997). *Tuesdays with Morrie: An old man, a young man, and life's greatest lesson*, New York: Doubleday.

American Psychiatric Association (2000) *Diagnostic and statistical manual of mental disorders* (4th ed., text revision). Washington, DC: American Psychiatric Association.

Barlow, D.H. (2002). *Anxiety and its disorders*. New York: The Guilford Press.

Bourne, E.J. (2005). *Anxiety and phobia workbook*. Oakland, CA: New Harbinger Publications.

Brantley, J. (2003). *Calming your anxious mind: How mindfulness and compassion can free you from anxiety fear and panic.* Oakland, CA: New Harbinger Publications.

Bronson, P. (2002). *What should I do with my life?: The true story of people who answered the ultimate question.* New York: Random House.

Broyard, A. (1992). *Intoxicated by my illness: And other writings on life and death,* New York: C. Potter.

Campbell, R.J. (1996). *Psychiatric dictionary* (7th ed.) Oxford: Oxford University Press.

de Botton, A. (2004). *Status anxiety.* New York: Pantheon Books.

Ellenberger, H. (1970). *The discovery of the unconscious: The history and evolution of dynamic psychiatry.* New York: Basic Books.

Elliott, C.H., & Smith, L.L. (2003). *Overcoming anxiety for dummies.* New York: Wiley Publishing, Inc.

Epstein, M. (1995). *Thoughts without a thinker: Psychotherapy from a Buddhist perspective.* New York: Basic Books.

Epstein, M. (1998). *Going to pieces without falling apart: A Buddhist perspective on wholeness.* New York: Broadway Books.

Frank, J.D., & Frank, J.B. (1991). *Persuasion and healing: A comparative study of psychotherapy* (3rd ed.) Baltimore, MD: Johns Hopkins University Press.

Freud, A. (1946). *The ego and the mechanisms of defence.* New York: International Universities Press, Inc.

Freud, S. (1959) Inhibitions, Symptoms and Anxiety, (1926 (1925)). In Strachey, J. (Vol. Ed.), *The standard edition of the complete psychological works of Sigmund Freud.* Vol. 20 (pp. 77–178). London: The Hogarth Press and the Institute of Psycho-Analysis.

Freud, S. (1959). Remembering, repeating, working through. In Strachey, J. (Vol. Ed.), *The standard edition of the complete psychological works of Sigmund Freud.* Vol. 12 (pp. 145–56). London: The Hogarth Press and the Institute of Psycho-Analysis.

Gabbard, G.O. (2000). *Psychodynamic psychiatry and clinical practice* (3rd ed.) Washington, DC: American Psychiatric Press, Inc.

Goleman, D. (2000). Emotional Intelligence. In Sadock, B.J., & Sadock, V.A. (Eds.), *Kaplan and Sadock's comprehensive textbook of psychiatry*, Vol. 1. Philadelphia: Lippincott Williams & Wilkins.

Herman, J. (1997). *Trauma and recovery.* New York: Basic Books.

Horowitz, M.J. (1999). *Essential papers on posttraumatic stress disorder.* New York: New York University Press.

Leary, M.R., & Kowalski, R.M. (1995). *Social anxiety.* New York: The Guilford Press.

LeDoux, J. (1996). *The emotional brain: The mysterious underpinnings of emotional life.* New York: Simon & Schuster.

Moyers, B. (1993). *Healing and the mind.* New York: Doubleday Books.

Nesse G.W., & Williams G.C. (1994). *Why we get sick: The new science of Darwinian medicine.* New York: Times Books.

Ratey, J., & Hallowell, E. (1994). *Driven to distraction.* New York: Pantheon Books.

Sadock, B.J., & Sadock, V.A. (Eds.). (2000). *Kaplan and Sadock's comprehensive textbook of psychiatry*, Vol. 1 (Anxiety disorders sections, pp. 1441–1503). Philadelphia: Lippincott Williams & Wilkins.

   a. Gorman, J.M. Introduction and overview, p. 1441.

   b. Horwath, E., & Weissman, M.M., pp. 1441–49.

   c. Sullivan, G.M., & Coplan, J.D. Biochemical aspects, pp. 1450–56.

   d. Fyer, A.J. Genetics, pp. 1457–1463.

   e. Gabbard, G.O. Psychodynamic aspects, pp. 1464–75.

   f. Pine, D.S. Clinical Features, pp. 1476–89.

   g. Papp, L.A. Somatic treatment, pp. 1490–97.

   h. Welkowitz, L.A. Psychological treatments, pp. 1498–1503.

Schmidt, M.D., Leonard J., & Warner, B. (2002). *Panic: Origins, insight, and treatment.* Berkeley, CA: North Atlantic Books.

Schwartz, J.M., with Beyette, B. (1996). *Brain lock: A four-step self-treatment method to change your brain chemistry.* New York: Regan Books.

Resources

175

Shengold, L. (1989). *Soul murder: The effects of childhood abuse and deprivation.* New Haven, CT: Yale University Press.

Stahl, S.M. (1996). *Essential psychopharmacology: Neuroscientific basis and practical applications.* Cambridge, MA: Cambridge University Press.

Vaillant, G. (1995). *Adaptation to life.* Cambridge, MA: Harvard University Press.

Vaughan, S.C. (1997). *The talking cure: The science behind psychotherapy.* New York: GP Putnam's Sons.

Organizations

American Psychiatric Association
1000 Wilson Boulevard
Suite 1825
Arlington, VA 22209
Tel. 703-907-7300
www.psych.org

American Psychoanalytic Association
309 E. 49th Street
New York, NY 10017
Tel. 212-752-0450
centraloffice@apsa.org

American Psychological Association
750 First Street, NE
Washington, DC 20002
Tel. 202-336-5500
www.apa.org

Anxiety Disorders Association of America
8730 Georgia Avenue, Suite 600
Silver Spring, MD 20910, USA
Tel. 240-485-1001
www.adaa.org

National Alliance for the Mentally Ill (NAMI)
Colonial Place Three
2107 Wilson Boulevard, Suite 300
Arlington, VA 22201
Tel. 703-524-7600
www.nami.org

**National Institute of Mental Health Information Resources
and Inquiries Branch**
(301) 443-4513

National Self-Help Clearinghouse
25 West 43rd Street
New York, NY 10036
(212) 354-8525

Resources

Rating Scales

Anxiety Disorders Self-Test for Family Members
How much anxiety is too much? Ask a family member to answer "yes" or "no" to the following questions by circling the appropriate answer next to each question; show the results to your health-care professional.

How can I tell if it's an anxiety disorder?
Yes or No? Are you troubled by:

Yes No   Repeated, unexpected panic attacks, during which you suddenly are overcome by intense fear or discomfort for no apparent reason, or the fear of having another panic attack?

Yes No   Persistent, inappropriate thoughts, impulses or images that you can't get out of your mind (such as a preoccupation with getting dirty, worry about the order of things, or aggressive or sexual impulses)?

Yes No   Powerful and ongoing fear of social situations involving unfamiliar people?

Yes No   Excessive worrying, for six months or more, about a number of events or activities?

Yes No   Fear of places or situations where getting help or escape might be difficult, such as in a crowd or on a bridge?

Yes No   Shortness of breath or a racing heart for no apparent reason?

Yes No   Persistent and unreasonable fear of an object or situation, such as flying, heights, animals, blood, etc.?

Yes No   Being unable to travel alone?

Yes No   Spending too much time each day doing things over and over again (for example, hand-washing, checking things, or counting)?

More days than not, do you:

Yes No   Feel restless?

Yes No   Feel easily tired distracted?

Yes No   Feel irritable?

Yes No   Have tense muscles or problems sleeping?

Yes No   Have you experienced or witnessed a traumatic event that involved actual or threatened death or serious injury to yourself or a loved one (for example, military combat, a violent crime or a serious car accident)?

Yes No   Does your anxiety interfere with your daily life?

Having more than one illness at the same time can make it difficult to diagnose and treat the different conditions. Illnesses that sometimes complicate anxiety disorders include depression and substance abuse. With this in mind, please take a minute to answer the following questions:

Yes No   Have you experienced changes in sleeping or eating habits?

More days than not, do you feel:

Yes No   Sad or depressed?

Yes No   Disinterested in life?

Yes No   Worthless or guilty?

During the last year, has the use of alcohol or drugs:

Yes No   Resulted in your failure to fulfill responsibilities with work, school, or family?

Yes No   Placed you in a dangerous situation, such as driving a car under the influence?

Yes No   Gotten you arrested?

Yes No   Continued despite causing problems for you and/or your loved ones?

If you or someone you know would like more information on helping a family member, please go to the ADAA resource page at *www.adaa.org*.

Generalized Anxiety Disorder (GAD) Self-Test[1]

How much anxiety is too much? If you suspect that you might suffer from generalized anxiety disorder, complete the following self-test by circling "yes" or "no" next to each question, and showing the results to your health-care professional.

How can I tell if it's GAD?

Yes or No? Are you troubled by:

Yes No   Excessive worry, occurring more days than not, for a least six months?

Yes No   Unreasonable worry about a number of events or activities, such as work or school and/or health?

Yes No   The inability to control the worry?

Are you bothered by any of the following?

Yes No   Restlessness, feeling keyed up or on edge?

Yes No   Being easily tired?

Yes No   Problems concentrating?

Yes No   Irritability?

Yes No   Muscle tension?

Yes No   Trouble falling asleep or staying asleep, or restless and unsatisfying sleep?

Yes No   Does your anxiety interfere with your daily life?

Having more than one illness at the same time can make it difficult to diagnose and treat the different conditions. Illnesses that sometimes complicate anxiety disorders include depression and substance abuse. With this in mind, please take a minute to answer the following questions:

Yes No   Have you experienced changes in sleeping or eating habits?

More days than not, do you feel:

Yes No   Sad or depressed?

Yes No   Disinterested in life?

Yes No   Worthless or guilty?

During the last year, has the use of alcohol or drugs:

Yes No   Resulted in your failure to fulfill responsibilities with work, school, or family?

Yes No   Placed you in a dangerous situation, such as driving a car under the influence?

Yes No   Gotten you arrested?

Yes No   Continued despite causing problems for you and/or your loved ones?

If you or someone you know would like more information on generalized anxiety disorders, please go to the ADAA resource page on this topic at *www.adaa.org*.

Obsessive Compulsive Disorder (OCD)[1,2]
If you suspect obsessive-compulsive disorder (OCD), the first step toward regaining control of your life is to seek help. Answer "yes" or "no" to the following questions by circling the appropriate answer, and show the test to your health-care professional at your first visit.

Could it be OCD?

Yes or No?

Yes No   Do you have unwanted ideas, images, or impulses that seem silly, nasty, or horrible?

Yes No   Do you worry excessively about dirt, germs, or chemicals?

Yes No   Are you constantly worried that something bad will happen because you forgot something important, like locking the door or turning off appliances?

Yes No   Do you experience shortness of breath?

Yes No   Are you afraid you will act or speak aggressively when you really don't want to?

Yes No   Are you always afraid you will lose something of importance?

Yes No   Are there things you feel you must do excessively or thoughts you must think repeatedly in order to feel comfortable?

Yes No   Do you have "jelly" legs?

Yes No   Do you wash yourself or things around you excessively?

Yes No   Do you have to check things over and over again or repeat them many times to be sure they are done properly?

Yes No   Do you avoid situations or people you worry about hurting by aggressive words or deeds?

Yes No   Do you keep many useless things because you feel that you can't throw them away?

Having more than one illness at the same time can make it difficult to diagnose and treat the different conditions. Illnesses that sometimes complicate an anxiety disorder include depression and

Rating Scales

substance abuse. With this in mind, please take a minute to answer the following questions:

Yes No   Have you experienced changes in sleeping or eating habits?

More days than not, do you feel:

Yes No   Sad or depressed?

Yes No   Disinterested in life?

Yes No   Worthless or guilty?

During the last year, has the use of alcohol or drugs:

Yes No   Resulted in your failure to fulfill responsibilities with work, school, or family?

Yes No   Placed you in a dangerous situation, such as driving a car under the influence?

Yes No   Gotten you arrested?

Yes No   Continued despite causing problems for you and/or your loved ones?

Panic Disorder Self-Test[1]

If you suspect you may be suffering from panic disorder, complete the following self-test by circling "yes" or "no" next to each question. Show the results to your health-care professional.

How can I tell if it's panic disorder?

Yes or no? Are you troubled by:

Yes No   Repeated, unexpected "attacks" during which you suddenly are overcome by intense fear or discomfort, for no apparent reason?

If yes, during this attack, did you experience any of these symptoms?

Yes No   Pounding heart

Yes No   Sweating

Yes No   Trembling or shaking

Yes No   Shortness of breath

Yes No   Choking

Yes No   Chest pain

Yes No   Nausea or abdominal discomfort

Yes No   "Jelly" legs

Yes No   Dizziness

Yes No   Feelings of unreality or being detached from yourself

Yes No   Fear of dying

Yes No   Numbness or tingling sensations

Yes No   Chills or hot flashes

Yes No   Do you experience a fear of places or situations where getting help or escape might be difficult, such as in a crowd or on a bridge?

Yes No   Does being unable to travel without a companion trouble you?

For at least one month following an attack, have you:

Yes No   Felt persistent concern about having another one?

Yes No   Worried about having a heart attack or going "crazy"?

Yes No   Changed your behavior to accommodate the attack?

Having more than one illness at the same time can make it difficult to diagnose and treat the different conditions. Illnesses that sometimes complicate an anxiety disorder include depression and substance abuse. With this in mind, please take a minute to answer the following questions:

Yes No   Have you experienced changes in sleeping or eating habits?

Rating Scales

185

More days than not, do you feel:

Yes No   Sad or depressed?

Yes No   Disinterested in life?

Yes No   Worthless or guilty?

During the last year, has the use of alcohol or drugs:

Yes No   Resulted in your failure to fulfill responsibilities with work, school, or family?

Yes No   Placed you in a dangerous situation, such as driving a car under the influence?

Yes No   Gotten you arrested?

Yes No   Continued despite causing problems for you and/or your loved ones?

Phobia Self-Test[1]
Phobias—illogical yet powerful fears—affect more than one in eight Americans at some time. Phobias are the most common kind of anxiety disorder. If you suspect that you might suffer from a phobia, complete the following self-test by circling "yes" or "no" next to each question. Show the results to your health-care professional.

How can I tell if it's a phobia?
Yes or no? Are you troubled by:

Yes No   Powerful and ongoing fear of social situations involving unfamiliar people?

Yes No   Fear of places or situations where getting help or escape might be difficult, such as in a crowd or on a bridge?

Yes No   Shortness of breath or a racing heart for no apparent reason?

Yes No   Persistent and unreasonable fear of an object or situation, such as flying, heights, animals, blood, etc.?

Yes No   Being unable to travel alone, without a companion?

Having more than one illness at the same time can make it difficult to diagnose and treat the different conditions. Illnesses that sometimes complicate anxiety disorders include depression and substance abuse. With this in mind, please take a minute to answer the following questions:

Yes No   Have you experienced changes in sleeping or eating habits?

More days than not, do you feel:

Yes No   Sad or depressed?

Yes No   Uninterested in life?

Yes No   Worthless or guilty?

During the last year, has the use of alcohol or drugs:

Yes No   Resulted in your failure to fulfill responsibilities with work, school, or family?

Yes No   Placed you in a dangerous situation, such as driving a car under the influence?

Yes No   Gotten you arrested?

Yes No   Continued despite causing problems for you and/or your loved ones?

Posttraumatic Stress Disorder Self-Test[1]
If you suspect that you might suffer from posttraumatic stress disorder, complete the following self-test by circling "yes or "no" next to each question. Show the results to your health-care professional.

How can I tell if it's PTSD?
Yes or No?

Yes No   Have you experienced or witnessed a life-threatening event that caused intense fear, helplessness or horror?

Do you reexperience the event in at least one of the following ways?

Yes No   Repeated, distressing memories and/or dreams?

Yes No   Acting or feeling as if the event were happening again (flashbacks or a sense of reliving it)?

Yes No   Intense physical and/or emotional distress when you are exposed to things that remind you of the event?

Do you avoid reminders of the event and feel numb, compared to the way you felt before, in three or more of the following ways:

Yes No   Avoiding thoughts, feelings, or conversations about it?

Yes No   Avoiding activities, places, or people who remind you of it?

Yes No   Blanking on important parts of it?

Yes No   Losing interest in significant activities of you life?

Yes No   Feeling detached from other people?

Yes No   Feeling your range of emotions is restricted?

Yes No   Sensing that your future has shrunk (for example, you don't expect to have a career, marriage, children, or a normal life span)?

Are you troubled by any of the following?

Yes No   Problems sleeping

Yes No   Irritability or outbursts of anger

Yes No   Problems concentrating

Yes No   Feeling "on guard"

Yes No   An exaggerated startle response

Having more than one illness at the same time can make it difficult to diagnosis and treat the different conditions. Illnesses that sometimes complicate an anxiety disorder include depression and substance abuse. With this in mind, please take a minute to answer the following questions:

Yes No   Have you experienced changes in sleeping or eating habits?

More days than not, do you feel:

Yes No   Sad or depressed?

Yes No   Disinterested in life?

Yes No   Worthless or guilty?

During the last year, has the use of alcohol or drugs:

Yes No   Resulted in your failure to fulfill responsibilities with work, school, or family?

Yes No   Placed you in a dangerous situation, such as driving a car under the influence?

Yes No   Gotten you arrested?

Yes No   Continued despite causing problems for you and/or your loved ones?

Social Phobia Self-Test[1]

Social phobia, or social anxiety disorder, affects more than 13% of Americans. It is a real and serious health problem that responds to treatment. The first step is seeking help. If you suspect that you might suffer from social phobia, complete the following self-test by circling "yes" or "no" next to each question. Show the results to your health-care professional.

How can I tell if it's social phobia?

Yes or no? Are you troubled by:

Yes No   An intense and persistent fear of a social situation in which people might judge you?

Yes No   Fear that you will be humiliated by your actions?

Rating Scales

189

Yes No   Fear that people will notice that you are blushing, sweating, trembling, or showing other signs of anxiety?

Yes No   Knowing that your fear is excessive or unreasonable?

Does the feared situation cause you to:

Yes No   Always feel anxious?

Yes No   Experience a "panic attack," during which you suddenly are overcome by intense fear or discomfort, including any of these symptoms?

Yes No   Pounding heart

Yes No   Sweating

Yes No   Trembling or shaking

Yes No   Shortness of breath

Yes No   Choking

Yes No   Chest pain

Yes No   Nausea or abdominal discomfort

Yes No   "Jelly" legs

Yes No   Dizziness

Yes No   Feelings of unreality or being detached from yourself

Yes No   Fear of losing control, "going crazy"

Yes No   Fear of dying

Yes No   Numbness or tingling sensations

Yes No   Chills or hot flashes

Yes No   Go to great lengths to avoid participating in the feared situation?

Yes No   Does all of this interfere with your daily life?

Having more than one illness at the same time can make it difficult to diagnose and treat the different conditions. Illnesses that sometimes complicate anxiety disorders include depression and substance abuse. With this in mind, please take a minute to answer the following questions:

Yes No   Have you experienced changes in sleeping or eating habits?

More days than not, do you feel:

Yes No   Sad or depressed?

Yes No   Disinterested in life?

Yes No   Worthless or guilty?

During the last year, has the use of alcohol or drugs:

Yes No   Resulted in your failure to fulfill responsibilities with work, school, or family?

Yes No   Placed you in a dangerous situation, such as driving a car under the influence?

Yes No   Gotten you arrested?

Yes No   Continued despite causing problems for you and/or your loved ones?

Anxiety Disorders in Adolescents: A Self-Test[1]

How much stress or worry is considered too much? Complete the following self-test by circling "yes" or "no" next to each question. Show the results to your health-care professional.

Is it an anxiety disorder?

Yes or No? As a teenager, are you troubled by:

Yes No   Repeated, unexpected "attacks" during which you suddenly are overcome by intense fear or discomfort for no apparent reason, or the fear of having another panic attack?

Rating Scales

191

Yes No   Persistent, inappropriate thoughts, impulses or images that you can't get out of your mind (such as a preoccupation with getting dirty or worry about the order of things)?

Yes No   Distinct and ongoing fear of social situations involving unfamiliar people?

Yes No   Excessive worrying about a number of events or activities?

Yes No   Fear of places or situations where getting help or escape might be difficult, such as in a crowd or on an elevator?

Yes No   Shortness of breath or racing heart for no apparent reason?

Yes No   Persistent and unreasonable fear of an object or situation, such as flying, heights, animals, blood, etc.?

Yes No   Being unable to travel alone, without a companion?

Yes No   Spending too much time each day doing things over and over again (for example, hand-washing, checking things, or counting)?

More days than not, do you:

Yes No   Feel restless?

Yes No   Feel easily fatigued or distracted?

Yes No   Experience muscle tension or problems sleeping?

More days than not, do you feel:

Yes No   Sad or depressed?

Yes No   Disinterested in life?

Yes No   Worthless or guilty?

Yes No   Have you experienced changes in sleeping or eating habits?

Yes No   Do you relive a traumatic event through thoughts, games, distressing dreams, or flashbacks?

Yes No   Does your anxiety interfere with your daily life?

Anxiety Disorders in Children: A Test for Parents[1]
If you think your child may have an anxiety disorder, please answer the following questions "Yes" or "No". Show the results to your child's health-care professional:

Yes No   Does the child have a distinct and ongoing fear of social situations involving unfamiliar people?

Yes No   Does the child worry excessively about a number of events or activities?

Yes No   Does the child experience shortness of breath or a racing heart for no apparent reason?

Yes No   Does the child experience age-appropriate social relationships with family members and other familiar people?

Yes No   Does the child often appear anxious when interacting with her peers and avoid them?

Yes No   Does the child have a persistent and unreasonable fear of an object or situation, such as flying, heights, or animals?

Yes No   When the child encounters the feared object or situation, does he react by freezing, clinging, or having a tantrum?

Yes No   Does the child worry excessively about her competence and quality of performance?

Yes No   Does the child cry, have tantrums, or refuse to leave a family member or other familiar person when she must?

Yes No   Has the child experienced a decline in classroom performance, refused to go to school, or avoided age-appropriate social activities?

Rating Scales

Yes No Does the child spend too much time each day doing things over and over again (for example, hand-washing, checking things, or counting)?

Yes No Does the child have exaggerated fears of people or events (e.g., burglars, kidnappers, car accidents) that might be difficult, such as in a crowd or on an elevator?

Yes No Does the child experience a high number of nightmares, headaches, or stomachaches?

Yes No Does the child repetitively reenact with toys scenes from a disturbing event?

Yes No Does the child redo tasks because of excessive dissatisfaction with less-than-perfect performance?

References

1. American Psychiatric Association. (1994). *Diagnostic and Statistical Manual of Mental Disorders* (4th ed.) Washington, DC: American Psychiatric Association.

2. Goodman, W.K., Price, L.H., et al. (1989). The Yale-Brown obsessive compulsive scale (Y-BOCS): Part 1. Development, use and reliability. *Arch Gen Psychiatry. 46*, 1006–1011.

Glossary

ADHD: *A*ttention *d*eficit/*h*yperactivity *d*isorder. A psychiatric disorder, more often in childhood, that involves a spectrum of inattentive symptoms (such as trouble paying attention or finishing projects) and/or hyperactive symptoms (such as an inability to sit still or impulsive behavior). While most people have some of these symptoms, those with actual ADHD find that it significantly interferes with their life.

Aggression: A natural human emotion that involves angry, sometimes violent, ideas or behaviors.

Agoraphobia: A fear of open spaces or places from which escape might be difficult or help unavailable.

Amygdala: A part of the limbic system of the brain that is involved with learning, coordination of sensory input, and emotions.

Antidepressant: A psychiatric medication that is used to treat not only depression, but a wide range of anxiety symptoms as well. There are numerous classes of these medications, each with its own mechanism of action and set of side effects.

Antipsychotic: A psychiatric medication that is used to treat psychosis (such as hearing voices or paranoia), as well as severe anxiety. These kinds of medications can also be helpful in small doses for sleep disorders, depression, and anxiety.

Anxiolytic: A psychiatric medication that is used to help control anxiety. There are several types of these medications, some to treat the acute symptoms of a panic attack and others to help stabilize anxiety over a longer period of time.

Attachment: The process of bonding to another human being during the course of development. Usually, one attaches first to his or her primary caregivers (e.g., parents) and then to other important people in his or her life. Attachment that is too strong can lead to separation anxiety, and attachment that is too weak can lead to difficulty with intimacy.

Benzodiazepine: A type of medication used to treat anxiety. Common medications include clonazepam, lorazepam, diazepam, and alprazolam. They have the potential to become addictive and have potentially dangerous withdrawal symptoms if taken in large doses.

Biofeedback: A method of monitoring one's physical responses to anxiety-inducing situations and attempting to lower the anxiety by reducing the physical response.

Computerized Axial Tomography (CAT) scan: An image of the body, such as the brain, that shows the anatomy of the brain tissue and can quickly identify masses or bleeding in the brain. It is relatively simple and involves only a few minutes in the actual scanner.

CBT: *C*ognitive *b*ehavioral *t*reatment. A form of psychotherapy that has been proven to be particularly helpful in anxiety and depression. It involves the identification of thoughts that may be unrealistic or untrue (e.g., "If I fail this test, my parents won't love me") and then coming up with alternative thoughts (e.g., "If I fail this test, my parents might be disappointed, but I tried my hardest and that is the best I can do") and behaviors.

Compulsion: A behavior, such as washing one's hands multiple times an hour, in response to an obsessive thought. Usually, the compulsion is done in order to alleviate the anxiety associated with the thought.

Conscious: Thinking that is in one's awareness. All thoughts, feelings, and behaviors that one is aware of thinking, feeling or doing, are conscious in contradistinction to unconscious.

Cortisol: A hormone secreted by the adrenal gland (a small gland on top of each kidney) in response to stressful situations, including anxiety, fear, excitement and physical stress.

Defense mechanism: A method of preventing harmful emotions from being felt. Defense mechanisms can be conscious, such as using humor to deal with a tragic situation, or unconscious, such as working excessively in order to avoid a painful situation at home.

Denial: A particular defense mechanism that involves a refusal to believe that something is true. This is outside of the person's control. For example, a woman who just learned that her son was arrested may use denial as a way to fend off her anger with and disappointment in her son, choosing instead to believe that the officers apprehended the wrong man.

Depression: A mood state in which one has numerous symptoms, including sleep and appetite disturbances, a decrease in energy level, concentration and interest, a feeling of sadness or isolation, and sometimes, thoughts of suicide. Depression is often accompanied by anxious symptoms. While most people feel "depressed" every now and then for a day or two, serious depression involves several weeks of these symptoms that significantly affect one's functioning.

DNA: *D*eoxyribo*n*ucleic *a*cid. The building block of all living creatures, it is a helical arrangement of proteins that carries one's genetic code.

D. O.: Doctor of Osteopathy. The degree that physicians who study osteopathy, or a system of medicine that studies the effects of the musculo-skeletal system on the rest of the body, obtain after four years of medical school.

DSM: The *Diagnostic and Statistical Manual* (now in its fourth edition). This book contains a listing of all of the identified psychiatric diagnoses and their symptoms. It is used by mental health care professionals to help diagnose and treat patients and to communicate with other professionals in the field.

Dysmorphia: The idea that one's body (or parts of one's body) looks much worse or deformed than it actually is.

EEG: *E*lectro*en*cephalogram. This is a kind of brain imaging technique, involving electrodes placed around the scalp, that measures brain waves and can detect abnormalities like seizures.

Ego: One of three theoretical parts of the mind, first established by Sigmund Freud, that involves a person's ability to interact with reality, regulate mood, and participate in normal daily interactions. The other two parts are the id and the superego.

Fear: An uncomfortable state of feeling, associated with anxiety, that something bad will or might happen.

Flashbacks: A phenomenon, usually seen in post-traumatic stress disorder (PTSD), in which a person has the sensation of reexperiencing a particular trauma. During the flashback, the person genuinely believes that he/she is being traumatized and is not aware of his/her real surroundings.

GABA: *G*amma-*a*mino*b*utyric *a*cid. A neurotransmitter in the central nervous system that is primarily involved in inhibiting impulses. This is the chemical that keeps excitatory neurotransmitters, like ones that cause anxiety, from getting out of control.

Genes: Packets of DNA, located on the chromosomes in each living cell of the human body, that carry all the information about how any given cell is supposed to function. Information is inherited from a parent to an off-spring through genes.

Genotype: The particular set of genes that a person has for a particular trait or feature. For example, the genotype for blue eyes is the set of genes that codes for that eye color. The actual blue color is called the phenotype, or how the genotype is represented.

Grief: A process during which a person mourns the loss of something, whether that be a loved one, a home, or even something less tangible, like self-esteem. If grief persists for a long time or becomes very serious, it can turn into depression.

Guilt: A feeling that one has done something wrong. Often accompanied by the feeling that one should be punished.

Hypnosis: A form of therapy in which a therapist induces a patient into an enhanced state of relaxation, possibly allowing for deeper memories or feelings to surface. This technique has been questioned recently in courts because of the propensity for people to be suggestible under hypnosis and possibly remember "false memories."

Hypochondriasis: An exaggerated fear that one has an illness or disease based on a misinterpretation of a bodily symptom and without any medical basis. For example, one may think that he has a brain tumor because he has a headache.

IBS: *Irritable bowel syndrome.* A group of symptoms, often associated with anxiety and more frequently found in women, that involves abdom-inal pain, constipation, diarrhea, and other gastrointestinal complaints without any clear medical reason.

Id: One of three theoretical parts of the mind, first established by Sigmund Freud, that represents a person's primal urges, such as sexual and aggressive impulses. The id is theoretically kept in control by the conscience, or the superego.

Imaging: The process of looking at parts of the human body that cannot be seen from the outside. Examples include x-rays, CAT scans and MRIs.

Insomnia: Difficulty with or an inability to sleep at night. Insomnia can involve trouble falling asleep, waking up too early and not being able to fall back asleep, or multiple awakenings during the night. Generally, people are then tired the next day. Associated with anxiety, depression, drug abuse, and medical conditions.

Limbic system: The part of the brain that controls emotional responses and experiences.

LPN: *Licensed practical nurse.* A basic-level nurse who has at least one year of training and has passed a state-administered licensing exam. LPNs are often supervised by an RN.

Masochism: A style of thinking and behavior that involves a desire, either conscious or unconscious, to be punished or to be submissive to another. While many people associate this term only with sexual activity, it can also apply to people who take on more work than they can handle, who push themselves to unbelievable limits, or who have difficulty saying, "No."

MD: *M*edical *d*octor. The degree that all physicians attain after successfully completing four years of medical school.

Meditation: A process of deep relaxation and intense focus, originated in India, during which contentment, decreased physical tension, and reduced anxiety are attained.

Mindfulness: A state of being aware of all of the details of one's surroundings. This technique is often used as a way to reach a state of meditation or relaxation.

Mood stabilizer: A psychiatric medication that is used to balance mood states. Mood stabilizers are particularly helpful in bipolar disorder (manic-depression) to prevent severe depression or dangerous manias.

MRI: *M*agnetic *r*esonance *i*maging. A type of imaging in which parts of the body, such as the brain, are visualized in much more detail than on a CAT scan. The process of an MRI involves lying in a narrow tube for up to an hour; this can be difficult for people with claustrophobia.

Neurochemistry: The study of the mechanisms and chemical components of the nervous system, including brain structure and neurotransmitter function.

Neurosis: A state of mental functioning often associated with anxiety, either conscious or unconscious, that does not significantly impair reality testing or one's personality. In its most basic sense, neurosis means responding to present stimuli with prior expectations.

Neurotransmitter: A chemical messenger in the nervous system that carries a message from one neuron to the next. Examples include serotonin and norepinephrine.

Norepinephrine: A neurotransmitter (chemical) that helps regulate mood and other physical symptoms of anxiety.

Obsession: A repetitive, intrusive thought that is difficult for one to get rid of, despite a knowledge that the thought is unreasonable. Sometimes obsessions can be relieved by compulsions.

Panic attack: A severe anxiety attack that can last for several minutes to an hour, usually without any obvious trigger, that involves multiple symptoms, including extreme fear, trouble breathing, increased heart rate, sweating, and shakes.

Pathologic: This refers to any medical condition that is considered abnormal.

Pathophysiology: The mechanisms of disease processes in the body and the ways in which disease alters normal structure and function.

PhD: *D*octor of *P*hilosophy. This degree is attained after one successfully completes years of coursework and research in a particular field (including psychology or social work).

Phenotype: The physical representation of a particular genetic code (genotype). For example, blue eyes

199

are the phenotype of the genes encoding blue eye color.

Physiology: Having to do with normal functioning of body systems and organs.

Psychiatry/psychiatrist: The study, diagnosis, treatment, and prevention of mental illness and behavioral disorders. Psychiatrists are medical doctors (MDs) who study and practice psychiatry.

Psychoanalysis: A form of intensive psychotherapy, usually 4–5 times per week, conducted with the patient lying on the couch, facing away from the analyst. Psychoanalysis is designed to help a patient recognize and work through unconscious conflicts such as ambivalent feelings toward a loved one or difficulty attaining intimacy in relationships. Sigmund Freud was the pioneer of this practice.

Psychodynamics: The study and science of how the mind develops and how the various parts of the mind interact with and influence each other.

Psychology/psychologist: The study of behavior and the processes underlying behavior. Psychologists are those who specialize in the study of psychology and have acquired their PhDs.

Psychoneuroimmunology: The study of the ways in which the neurological immunological mental systems interface (for example, getting a cold during times of high stress).

Psychopharmacotherapy: The use of medication, prescribed by psychiatrists, to treat mental illness.

Psychosis: A state of thinking in which reality is distorted in a severe way. Examples would be hearing voices, experiencing paranoia that the FBI is following you, or an inability to link thoughts logically together. Psychosis can be caused by many things, including mental illness, drug abuse, and medical conditions.

Psychotherapy: A general term to describe many different types of psychological and psychiatric treatments that involve communication and talking between the patient and the therapist.

RN: *R*egistered *n*urse. A nurse who has 2–4 years of education and training and is responsible for basic and advanced nursing care.

Rumination: The process of going over and over the same thought in one's mind to the exclusion of other thoughts and without any clear benefit. Often a symptom of anxiety.

Sadism: A style of thinking and behavior that involves a desire, either conscious or unconscious, to punish or to be dominant over others. While many people associate this term only with sexual activity, it can also apply to people who are intentionally cruel without any apparent self-benefit.

Self-mutilation: The practice of injuring oneself, usually by cutting, burning, or piercing. The underlying etiology of such behavior can be varied, but some self-mutilate in an attempt to control inner feelings of emptiness; the pain associated with the mutilation helps one to feel "alive."

Serotonin: A neurotransmitter (chemical) in the central nervous system that is involved in many different activities, including motor function, mood regulation, and perception.

Shame: A feeling that accompanies the uncovering of humiliating or embarrassing thoughts or behaviors.

Somatization: A process by which a person expresses emotional discomfort, most commonly anxiety, in the form of somatic, or bodily, symptoms. For example, a person might complain of persistent abdominal pain in the face of an upcoming transition, without any medical explanation. Once the transition has stabilized, the abdominal pain may disappear.

SRI: *S*erotonin *r*euptake *i*nhibitor. A type of medication that is used to treat depression and anxiety by decreasing the rate at which serotonin is metabolized in the nervous system, resulting in higher concentrations of that neurotransmitter.

Stress: A general term to describe any event or situation that raises a person's anxiety.

Stimulant: A class of amphetamine-based medications that is used to treat ADHD and can sometimes help with the treatment of depression. Other stimulants that are not used for treatment include caffeine, nicotine, and cocaine.

Superego: Also known as the "conscience," one of three theoretical parts of the mind, first established by Sigmund Freud, that represents a person's internal moral compass. The superego keeps the impulses from the id in check so that a person can conform to societal, cultural, moral, and ethical expectations. The superego also helps regulate guilt.

TCM: *T*raditional *C*hinese *m*edicine.

Temperament: The style of interaction and attachment with which a person is naturally born. Some people are naturally easy going, while others are "slow to warm up."

TMJ: *T*emporo*m*andibular *j*oint. The joint that connects the jaw to the skull. This joint can become irritated and inflamed if a person grinds his or her teeth excessively or clenches his or her jaw, usually due to anxiety. The irritation can lead to pain and headaches.

Unconscious: The thought processes of which one is not aware. Dreams are a good representation of unconscious thoughts. One of the goals of psychoanalysis is to help the unconscious thoughts become conscious.

Index